Researching

Researching Older People's Nursing

The Gap between Theory and Practice

Christine Smith

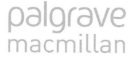

First published 2010 by
PALGRAVE MACMILLAN

Palgrave Macmillan in the UK is an imprint of Macmillan Publishers Limited,
registered in England, company number998, of Houndmills, Basingstoke,
Hampshire RG21 6XS.

Palgrave Macmillan in the US is a division of St Martin's Press LLC,
175 Fifth Avenue, New York, NY 10010.

Palgrave Macmillan is the global academic imprint of the above companies
and has companies and representatives throughout the world.

Palgrave® and Macmillan® are registered trademarks in the United States,
the United Kingdom, Europe and other countries

ISBN 978-0-230-51647-2

This book is printed on paper suitable for recycling and made from fully
managed and sustained forest sources. Logging, pulping and manufacturing
processes are expected to conform to the environmental regulations of the
country of origin.

A catalogue record for this book is available from the British Library.

10   9   8   7   6   5   4   3   2   1
19   18   17   16   15   14   13   12   11   10

Printed in Great Britain by CPI Antony Rowe, Chippenham and Eastbourne

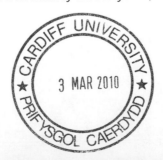

Contents

List of figures and tables   vi

Preface   vii

Foreword   ix

Acknowledgements   xii

Introduction   1

Part I: Research and theory   7

1 An ethnography of older people's nursing   9

2 Theory development in nursing   25

3 Building professional knowledge in older people's care   52

Part II: Research and practice   63

4 The context and culture of the care setting   65

5 A framework for the delivery of care   79

6 Focusing on the practice of caring for older people   111

7 Future trends: standards and quality in care   126

References   138

Index   149

List of figures and tables

Figures

2.1 The technical rationality model and its relationship
between theory and practice 31
2.2 Reflexive practice in action 41
2.3 The reflective cycle 44
4.1 Staff engaging with the long-term management of
older people 69
4.2 Aims of remodelling care of older people in primary
care 71
5.1 Themes and categories of caring for an older person
as seen in practice 80
5.2 Common features present in care of older people 81
5.3 Factors in caring for an older person 84
6.1 Informal practice theorising within older people's
nursing practice 117
7.1 Number of people aged 50 and over 131

Tables

1.1 Factor isolation: advising identified as a factor in the
theme of nutrition 22
2.1 Definitions of nursing theory 28

Preface

Political trends as well as changes in health needs have made care of older people top of the political agenda; this is the case not only for health but also social care. Nursing care of older people is an important part of primary and secondary care delivery, which plays a major role in the work of both hospital and community nurses. However, it has to be admitted that the majority of newly qualified nurses would not choose to work in this setting and have not always viewed care of older people as an area in which to develop their careers. As a result, care of older people has been called the 'Cinderella of nursing'.

The author's interest in the issue of practice theory arose from her work as a nurse lecturer in teaching nursing theory and, in particular, reflective practice with students on graduate study courses. During these courses nurses were encouraged, through reflective practice sessions in experiential workshops, to reflect on incidents from their own practice. 'Critical Incident Analysis' was developed using reflective frameworks to explore nurses' knowledge (Carper, 1978; Meizirow, 1990; Johns, 1996) that underpinned their practice. It seems that reflective practice has gained popularity within nurse education and practice, with the purpose of enabling practitioners to assess, understand and learn through their lived experience, and from this to develop awareness and increased effectiveness within their own nursing practice. Reflective practice is seen as a model for structured reflection on experience. Within this process any discrepancies between desirable practice and actual practice are made visible and became the focus of discussion and analysis. Essentially, learning in this way is by a process of enlightenment, empowerment and emancipation (Johns, 1996). It became evident to the author in the reflective practice sessions she experienced that the 'knowledge' recounted when describing practice was not as readily available or, importantly, the same as the knowledge found in the nursing textbooks or the nursing literature.

This led to a research interest in the comparison of practice theory and the actual knowledge used by nurses in practice. The author was made aware, through reflective practice teaching, that there was a difference in 'known' nursing theories and those taught. In relation to this, the work of Argyris and Schon (1974) has been increasingly pertinent to nurse teachers involved in teaching reflective practice. The contribution to their scholarship in terms of the differences between espoused theories (what the nurse says they do) and theories in use (what they actually do) has been significant in terms of nurse education. Rolfe et al. (2001) have argued that one of the problems for any practice-based discipline with accepting scientific knowledge as being dominant is that it implies a particular model of the relationship between knowledge and practice.

Schon alerted educationalists to the inadequacies of technical rationality and suggested that practitioners have to deal with problems as they arise in practice. Technical Rationality assumes that empirical science based on facts is the only source of knowledge and all problems in practice can be solved by scientific facts. Schon (1991) argued, however, that practice situations are characterised by complexity, uncertainty, instability, uniqueness and value conflicts. The author chose to research into the issue of practice-based knowledge in the care of older people because care of older people is a rich source of nursing input. The key purpose was to find out what information and theories nurses used in their everyday practice to base their practice on when caring for older people. Further discussion of the research and its findings can be found within this book.

In this book Christine Smith tackles a number of very important issues for all nurses. First, as she points out in her opening remarks, it is well known that many nurses do not want to work with the elderly. This point needs to be explored and is explored well in this book. The demographic fact is that the elderly population in the UK is increasing; those elderly people are also living longer. Such people will not only need care, they will need *good* care. This book is likely to be of great value to anyone who wants to explore these issues and to reflect on them – for the nature of this book is a reflective one. The researcher, by highlighting her own ability to reflect, also calls upon the reader to do the same.

For a number of years, the concepts of reflection and of caring in nursing have been highlighted. Many educators are keen to teach their students how to reflect on their practice and many nurses have gone on to use those skills in the practice arena. I confess to having some reservations about reflection – particularly after the event – as I doubt our ability to remember what we have done or what we have felt about a particular sequence or aspect of care. However, this book is an excellent advertisement for the value of all of the positive aspects of reflection.

Similarly, caring has long been identified as a core construct in nursing. It is particularly interesting that Dr Smith's respondents identified caring as a major aspect of their clinical work. This finding thus reinforces much of the theoretical literature that has gone before. The author has managed to convey the insights of her respondents without 'getting in the way' of what they have to say. The ethnographic element of this study is both educational and valuable to a wide range of nurses: from those setting out in the profession, to nurse researchers and to those in clinical practice. It is rare that one book can meet the needs of so many audiences in this way but I believe that this volume can.

What I find particularly excellent about this book is that it brings together two particular aspects of nursing that have often been separated: nursing theory and nursing practice. Given nursing's need to develop an academic knowledge base, early nursing theories (and also nursing models) were usually constructed without recourse to the theorists conducting research. This was thoroughly understandable. Nursing was fast becoming an academic discipline and academic disciplines need theories from which to draw. On the other hand, research takes time to do and time to build up into a body of knowledge. Thus, the early pioneers of academic nursing 'invented' their theories and models.

In Dr Smith's book, we find a very helpful marriage of theory and practice. She explores respondents' own theories about how they care for elderly people and then links these 'personal' theories to existing theory. In doing this, she achieves a number of things. First, she allows the reader to revisit nursing theories. Second, she makes transparent the way that nurses 'theorise' in real life. Third, she encourages a rethinking of many of the principles by which theory is constructed and of how care may be delivered.

The book makes clear the way in which the study was conducted. In this respect, it is a useful example to other researchers – both experienced and beginner. I have always felt that the best writing is clear and simple. Complicated concepts can easily be conveyed simply, when the writer gives it a little thought. Christine's book is an example of this. The fields of reflection, ethnography and caring are often represented by authors who feel the need to use big words and long sentences to convey what they have to say. It is refreshing to read a book in which this is not the case. Christine Smith's writing style is happily free of impenetrable prose.

This is a book written by a nurse, for other nurses. Anyone working with elderly people will benefit from reading it. Any nursing researcher will also find much here to help them with their work. Students will appreciate the sympathetic tone of the book and its insights into research, theory and care. The layout of the book, with its pull-out boxes of points for reflection, will help the reader to stop and ponder on each of the sections he or she has read.

The fact remains that all of us are getting older. One day, you, the reader, will be old. What sort of care will you want? In this field of nursing, perhaps more than any other, the Golden Rule should apply. We should treat others as we, ourselves, would want to be treated. This book will help you to consider and apply that rule.

Philip Burnard, PhD
Emeritus Professor of Nursing
Cardiff University, Wales, UK
2009

Acknowledgements

This book is dedicated to my son Tomas with love.

I would like to thank all the nurses working in care of older people who were involved with this study. These nurses agreed to be observed and interviewed and gave their time freely during times of staff shortages. Their trust and the discussion they provided were invaluable.

Many thanks to Professor Paul Wainwright for being very supportive, constructive and encouraging whilst I conducted my PhD study and wrote my thesis.

I would like to express my sincere thanks to the many colleagues who along the way have engaged with me in conversations and stimulating debates that have helped me to develop this work.

Thanks to Gail Sullivan, Angela Bowyer and Dr Michelle Huws-Thomas for their help and support and to the staff at Palgrave Macmillan, especially Lynda Thompson, Commissioning Editor.

Textual acknowledgements

Figure 2.2 is reproduced with the kind permission of Elsevier.
Figure 7.1 is reproduced with the kind permission of the controller of the Office of Public Sector Information.

Every effort has been made to trace all the copyright holders, but if any have been inadvertently overlooked the publishers will be pleased to make the necessary arrangement at the earliest opportunity.

Introduction

It is a well-known fact that student nurses don't always want to work with older people; with their lack of experience they cannot see what new technical skills they are going to acquire or achieve. The framework outlined in this book (see Chapter 5) offers a new insight into the complexities of practice and helps the reader to view nursing from a more nurturing, caring and supporting aspect of both primary and secondary care, highlighting the positive experiences and useful skills that nursing older people draws out.

We live in changing times in healthcare and the demand that practice should be evidence based requires nurses to be able to interpret, evaluate and apply published research in their everyday practice. This book advocates qualitative research methods which can be conducted by experienced nurses/practitioners to advance their knowledge in the future.

The main purpose of this book is to share the results of the author's original research, which identified the gap between nursing theory and nursing practice, specifically focusing on nurses caring for older people. It takes a practical perspective that attempts to articulate the complexity of caring for older people, which is often seen as mundane work. The heart of the book is centred on an approach to the care of older people based on a framework developed by the author (utilising ethnography as a research method). The framework gives direction to aspects of nursing practice that nurses value most in caring for older people. The framework has been developed straight from practice itself and hence it is hoped that it will be useful to nurses working in care of older people in order to help develop their own practice.

The original research study had two strands. The first was to explore what theories nurses used to give care in a practical situation. The second was to discover how nurses arrive at an 'answer' to deal with their patients' complex needs in their daily practice. The research showed that the care given by nurses is influenced by ongoing experiences, education in nursing and a range of social and political issues and psychological factors. There is a mass of knowledge available in policy documents, books and articles and these also act as triggers for professional responses in practice.

This book also demonstrates the main centrality of the purpose of the research, which was to develop an ethnography of the older person. Non-participant observation was undertaken on complete episodes of nursing practice, followed by semi-structured interviews to discuss the nursing care observed. The research data was analysed to generate categories and themes. A further process of factor isolation identified the practice theory in use. The practice theory isolated was about significant issues to the older person's wellbeing.

This work has shown that practical wisdom in older people's nursing is not always about scientific knowledge, since it is accomplished through an understanding of a particular situation with no two situations ever being the same. It acknowledges the nurses' informal practice knowledge not in theoretical propositions but as a reflectively processed repertoire of individual cases. Practical wisdom, in this stance, refers to the nurses' capacity to take the right course of action when faced with particular, complex situations which allow the practitioner to use general or universal theoretical knowledge. Informal theory has an important part to play in guiding and informing practice. Applying theory to practice involves some formal and some informal theory and is tailor-made to each practice situation. Practical knowledge in the context of individual situations cannot be universal, as with the product of grand theories or nursing models, because it cannot be taken away from the context in which that individual situation occurs. Each individual situation is unique, one of a kind. It is the nurse who employs his or her own professional judgement in order to decide the usefulness of research for practice.

In doing this study a vast amount of information was collected about what decisions nurses make in practical situations, and this gave a clear understanding of the sorts of issues that nurses are concerned about in their everyday work and the knowledge base for their actions. In addition to these, the issues that nurses talk about and value the most in their care delivery have been captured. This book is based on one research study; clearly, the information is not generalisable and as such the limitations of this are acknowledged. It does, however, give an insight into the work of nurses and decisions being made in caring for older people. It also offers a framework on which to base nursing practice. The study provides another piece of evidence for nurses to assess and inform their practice.

Outline of the book

Readership

This book is intended for post-registration nurses at various stages of their professional development. The book offers them the opportunity to read the idiosyncratic arguments reflecting the research base as the evidence on which to discuss nursing care of older people. To this end this book is less of a textbook than one would normally associate with studying nursing and rather a platform for debating current understandings of care of older people and research methods. It is not an attempt to provide an all-round book to cover just about everything on care of older people. Instead, it offers a unique and an individual approach with evidence-based nursing care which acknowledges the unique contribution both of the older person and the nurse. The author hopes that nurses reading the book enjoy it and take time to pause for thought on their everyday experiences.

The book will also be a useful resource for students studying either Ageing or Gerontological Nursing or for those studying ethnography as a research approach. As well as using the book as a supplementary text particularly within the area of health and social care, this book will also be of interest to multidisciplinary practitioners working in the field of care of older people.

Uniquely, this book considers the development of nursing theory for the care of older people and focuses on the developments in creation of nursing knowledge around care of older people. Given the changes in policy in care of older people with the publication of the National Service Guidelines and its particular emphasis on individual approaches to care, this book is essential reading for all. *Better Health in Old Age* (Department of Health [DoH], 2004) shows how the National Service Framework for older people has been important in modernising attitudes towards older people, and in shaping the approach to the organisation of health and social services.

This book will offer readers two main areas of nursing developments: nursing theory in relation to the older person, and a means of understanding ethnography as a methodological approach. With regard to nursing care of the older person, this book will offer a new way of looking at the development of nursing theory for care of older people and offers a unique area of knowledge relating to the practice theories of nurses in their everyday work in practice. The book proposes a framework and a new approach to working with older people.

Pause for thought

'Pause for thought' boxes have been added to the text to enable readers to take the time to look back on their experiences in nursing older people and to explore issues of caring for older people. The aim of these is to make time for readers to think about their own practice in terms of what issues influence the development of their practice experiences.

Layout of the book

Each chapter provides nurses with relevant sources and suggested reading that may be useful. These books either represent care of older people, or research or ethnography. As well as being focused towards the care of older people it is intended that post-registration nurses undertaking research will find this book a useful addition to the more theoretical-focused research-methods textbooks.

In the book the author has chosen primarily to use the term 'older people' although other terms such as 'patient', 'client' or 'service user' could be used.

Part I: Research and theory

Chapter 1

This chapter outlines how the author developed an ethnography of older people's nursing and gives an account of the research methodology of ethnography. The purpose of the research and how the understanding of this methodology is useful to the practice of nursing older people is also discussed.

Chapter 2

This chapter starts with what a theory is and the purpose of a theory; the different levels of theory and where they are derived from. An explanation of practice theory is given so that the reader is aware of its meaning in this text. Examples of mid-range theories are given as well as the differences between practice theory and other theories. The issue of practical wisdom is introduced and its contribution to professional practice is discussed. The benefits that can be obtained from developing a practice based on relevant theories and values are highlighted.

Chapter 3

Developing professional knowledge in caring for older people poses the fundamental questions of what is theory, and what theory is used and most valued by nurses. This chapter examines the role of research and formal knowledge in guiding practice and considers how the technical rationality model of formal science can be problematic when applying this in nursing practice.

Part II: Research and practice

Chapter 4

This chapter will look at the setting and environment for nursing older people in hospital in which the research study in this book was undertaken.

Chapter 5

This chapter discusses the framework that emerged from the author's research study. This chapter and the next focus on the application of the new framework.

Chapter 6

Chapter 6 looks at the various aspects of personalised care for older people. The framework presented provides a holistic approach to caring for older people which is unique in this field.

Chapter 7

This final chapter maps the author's strategies for moving forward. It looks at the care of older people in the future, considering global health issues and the challenges to be met in terms of how to achieve world-class standards for older people in key services. Nurses working with older people are key health professionals in encouraging healthy lifestyles, and integrated approaches to working will be discussed as well as creative and action-based nursing developments.

Part I

Research and theory

Chapter 1

An ethnography of older people's nursing

This chapter:

▶ discusses the development of an ethnography;
▶ discusses the research methodology for the study of older people in this book.

Developing research methods for the ethnography of older people

This book explores the practice-based theory of nurses working in older people's nursing with the intention of giving the reader a rich source of understanding of the practice theories of nurses working within this specialism. Practice theory is a relatively new subject in nursing and the purpose of using an exploratory qualitative approach was to gain an insight into what is going on and what factors are related to practice theory.

It explores what informal theories nurses use in caring for older people. The author answers this question through examining everyday experiences of nurses who care for older people. It seemed reasonable to visit the nurses in their working environment to observe and ask their views about what they did and why they did it.

The methodology was developed by the author to study what practice theories nurses use to base their everyday care on, and to look in more depth at the care of older people. A qualitative exploratory ethnographic research approach has the advantage of getting close to informal practice theory and would therefore have the potential to obtain a great deal of in-depth information about nursing care.

Several methodological challenges were used to explore the nature of the informal 'theory in use' of nurses working in the speciality of care of the older person. The study generated new knowledge by gaining meaning and understanding of the relationships of the informal practice theories identified:

▶ It explored the relationship between theory-in-use and the relevant literature.
▶ It explored the sources of knowledge which nurses draw upon in the practice of older adult nursing.
▶ It defined the factors and their relationships of informal theory in older people's nursing.

The aim of the research was to study nurses' meaning, behaviour and practice in the natural setting and to collect naturally occurring data in care of older people (Lincoln and Guba, 1985; Hammersley and Atkinson, 1995). Qualitative research describes in words, rather than numbers, the qualities of older people's nursing through observation and interviews. The advantages of using qualitative research over quantitative methods seemed clear in situations where there is little pre-existing knowledge, such as informal practice theory in nursing, and also where the issues are sensitive or complex (Benner, 1984; Lawler 1991; Meerabeau, 1992).

In 1995, Hammersley and Atkinson discussed the value of ethnography as a social research method based on cultural patterns and their existence for understanding social processes. Therefore, the author sought to understand the cultural perspective of nursing older people using observation, interviewing and field notes. Fieldwork is essential in ethnographic research and involves working with the nurses for long periods of time in the naturalistic setting – in this case, acute hospitalised settings. Ethnographic accounts identify the social complexities and explain social patterns of a group.

Ethnographic data collection methods were not regarded merely as a given set of research techniques but a process through which one could generate and interpret abstract views of the informal practice theory. The aim of the ethnographic approach was in a sense to explain the 'taken-for-granted' aspects of the work of nurses in the speciality of older people.

Ethical issues of researching care of older people

Ethical approval was sought from the local research ethics committee in the Health Authority. The author submitted a research proposal, a series of information sheets for patients and nurses, and consent forms.

All the nurses involved were given an explanation of the purpose of the research and both verbal and written consent was obtained. The nurses being observed were also required to gain permission and access from the patient and relatives. As a researcher, the author was able to observe daily activities from the viewpoint of a researcher and ethnographer. At all times the nurses were treated with respect and acknowledged as people with worthwhile experiences to share. Denzin and Lincoln (2005) advise that ethical research requires that there should be safeguards to protect the privacy and identity of research subjects. Identities, locations of individuals and places are concealed in published results, and data collected was held in anonymised form, and kept securely confidential.

The author was aware that ethical issues that arise are not just those of informed consent and confidentiality but also the manner in which the research is conducted in terms of safety aspects (Denzin and Lincoln, 2005). At times the author waited outside the room during intimate nursing activities and was able to explore this more fully in the interviews which followed. If, during the research, an emergency or other situation arose in which a patient's safety was at risk, the study would be stopped and the appropriate action taken until sufficient help arrived.

Sampling decisions

Sampling decisions were made at two levels: initial decisions had to be made about the group to be studied, followed by decisions about who and what was to be selected from within that group. This is what Hammersley and Atkinson (1995) referred to as 'sampling within the case'. Much qualitative research is carried out in a single setting, or with a small sample of nurses. Lincoln and Guba (1985) suggested that theoretical sampling may be ongoing throughout the research project, as the researcher seeks to develop and refine theoretical propositions which emerge from the data. The following methods of data collection were used in the study:

- ▶ Non-participant observation of a complete episode of practice was conducted.
- ▶ Field notes were written during the observation.

▶ Semi-structured interviews were conducted with those nurses observed in practice to clarify, ratify and explore the observations; also to identify the relevant knowledge.
▶ Questions were directly related to the care given as observed.
▶ A framework schedule was implemented, including cue questions, to identify the source of the 'theories in action'.
▶ Interviews were taped.
▶ Transcripts were returned to the nurses to be checked for accuracy.
▶ Research data was compared with the theoretical literature on care of older people.

All nurses who took part in this study were qualified Registered General Nurses (RGN) who had been working with older people for a minimum of one year. During the selection process no attempt was made to specifically select nurses of certain ages, backgrounds or gender. The nurse participants possessed various qualifications; some had undertaken post-registration courses, including modules relevant to working in older people's nursing. They all had varying degrees of experience that would be found in similar settings. Overall, the author conducted 40 observations and 40 interviews following those observations, and the data for the study was collected over a four-year period.

Methods, observations, interviews and field notes

The ethnographic approach to studying settings is derived from the anthropological tradition. Silverman (2006: 48) advises that 'the participant observer's aim is to take the viewpoint of those being studied, understanding the situated character of interaction'.

It was seen as important that the author had a clear idea about what was being observed. A single event within practice can entail a number of detailed activities and complex issues. No observer could absorb and record an indefinite number of details and so guidelines specifying the manner in which the observations were focused and documented were produced:

▶ Only one complete episode from practice was used for each practice session, and included several activities of nursing practice.
▶ The field notes included details about the observations but did not contain direct quotes and therefore were broadly interpretative.

▶ Each observation would be followed by a semi-structured interview to discuss the nursing practice observed.

The author did not explore the nursing practice in a task-centred way by choosing an intervention; the aim instead was to capture the total remit of nursing care. It was seen as being important that each episode of care had a beginning and end point to avoid any saturation of data collection by the author and to ensure that the focus was on one episode of care at any one time. Box 1.1 shows an example of some of the clinical work that was being performed:

Box 1.1　Episodes of care observed

▶ Admission of patients
▶ Discharge of patients
▶ Feeding and nutrition
▶ Dressing and grooming
▶ Hygiene needs
▶ Assessment of the patient
▶ Communication with patients and relatives
▶ Elimination
▶ Mobilising and rehabilitation
▶ Moving and turning patients
▶ Aseptic techniques and applying sterile dressings
▶ Medication and pain control

The author chose the role of an 'observer', which provided the freedom to observe and interview with minimal impact on the work role. Choosing not to participate in nursing activities was agreed as it was felt that this would impinge on the primary role of collecting data and would also influence what the nurses did in their nursing. For each observation session, it was hoped that an accurate record of what was happening would be obtained and this was then followed up by a semi-structured interview. The interview allowed the author to explore the reasons for the nurse's actions and to ratify the sources of knowledge (Lincoln and Guba, 1985).

The author observed practice at different times of the day to account for the shift patterns and this also helped to gain a better overview of practice throughout the daytime. Each conducted observation of nurses giving holistic care to patients lasted no longer than two hours. In order to establish a complete picture of care being delivered the data was collected in half-shifts during the morning or afternoon. The involvement of an observer has been questioned and has given rise to concerns about the potential reactivity of observational studies – that if the nurses had any knowledge that they were involved in research, this could be sufficient to alter their reactions. The author was aware that the prolonged engagement in this study was likely to reduce such reactive effects. As in any clinical setting, the *need* for practitioners to carry out their practice is likely to reduce reactivity. It was made clear to the nurses at the beginning of the shift that the purpose of the visit was to collect data and that the only intervention would be to reply to a patient when spoken to: for example, passing items from the locker if requested or, if the need arose, calling for help in an emergency.

Whilst the author conducted observations in the clinical area a white coat was worn, with an identification badge stating 'Nurse Researcher', ensuring that the purpose for being in the clinical situation was visible. An informal manner was intended to ensure comfort to those being observed and to make her presence as unobtrusive as possible, although the author was aware of the presence effect described as reactivity and observer interference (Denzin and Lincoln, 2005), as discussed above.

Establishing rapport is a key factor in observational research and there should be good interaction between the nurses and the researcher. The purpose and nature of the research was shared with the staff and the author defined her role as one of researcher and non-participant. There did not appear to be any objections to this research; in fact the nurses seemed interested in the topic of practice theory.

In order to prevent the possibility of the nurses 'getting ready', an appointment schedule for the purpose of the data collection was not implemented and the author retained the freedom to enter and leave the ward area as and when required. A pilot study was undertaken as a trial run of the methodology and time was spent detecting any problems in the method for gathering data.

Interviews of nurses

The decision was made to use semi-structured interviews. Although each interview covered a core of questions relating to sources of knowledge informing the nurses' practice, the semi-structured format allowed for any other issues to be raised spontaneously by the nurses. A semi-structured interview schedule was developed using the observation data and ideas from the literature, and was previously tested in the pilot study. The schedule contained brief headings for each of the issues to be discussed, which acted as an aide-memoire rather than a prescriptive instrument. It was not intended in any way to achieve uniformity or to prevent nurses from taking the initiative to let their experiences be known. Through this research method the author gained the trust and confidence of those being interviewed. The use of semi-structured interviews enabled the author to create a safe environment in which the viewpoints and personal experiences of the nurses could be actively sought.

Hammersley and Atkinson (1995) considered it essential to allow uninterrupted time for interviews and the author of this study set aside 30–45 minutes per interview. Nurses were reminded of their right to withdraw from the study at any time and their right to refuse to answer questions during the interview. It was also made clear to them that the data used and recorded would be done so only with their full knowledge and consent.

Throughout the interviews the author made sure that the language used was easy to understand and jargon free and that all interviews were audio-taped. The tape recorder was invaluable, sensitively used and accepted by the nurses. The advantage in recording information in this way was that repeatedly replaying the tapes allowed the author to capture the particular meaning of what was being said. It also allowed the author to be free from the task of writing copious notes, better able to concentrate on the nurses' accounts and watch for non-verbal as well as verbal responses in following up answers (Silverman, 2006).

The interviews were transcribed from the tape recordings as soon as possible after the interviews in order to establish that the transcripts represented an accurate picture of what took place in the interviews. These transcripts were then returned to each nurse to confirm their accuracy. This proved to be extremely useful and the nurses were also pleased to see that the author spent time on the details of the research and showed concern for them and their nursing practice.

Field notes consisted of the jotting down of salient points that were reworked in detail later the same day. They took the form of reconstruction of interactions, short conversation extracts or description of events (Lincoln and Guba, 1985). Field notes were written during the observations of nursing care and also when the nurses were writing their care plans.

Researcher reflexivity

Reflexivity should be seen as a continuous process of reflection by the individual researcher on their own values, preconceptions, behaviour or presence and those of the nurses, which can affect responses (Hammersley and Atkinson, 1995). Qualitative research emphasises the embedding of research data in the circumstances of the research settings. The analysis of research data should therefore involve careful reflection upon the ways in which the research process has shaped the data itself. The author felt that such reflexivity would also take account of her own prior personal biases and recognise the roles and values of these in the development of the research findings. Reflexivity implies that the orientation will be shaped by the research work, including the value and interest of the research locations. The importance of linking the analysis of qualitative research data to the circumstances of the research process relates then to reflexivity (Hammersley and Atkinson, 1995). Qualitative research accounts for self-conscious reflection upon the ways in which the findings of the research are inevitably shaped by the research process and the analysis should account for this.

'Going native' is also recognised as an aspect of spending a prolonged period of time in the research setting. Without realising it, the researcher may begin to share the assumptions of the nurses. This problem may arise, for example, where decisions made by the nurses were based on assumptions shared by the author and she may have been unable to gain sufficient distance to treat these assumptions as problematic.

In the quantitative tradition the emphasis is upon eliminating the impact of research upon the findings. The credibility of research is strengthened when the researcher can demonstrate that both data collection and analysis are considered by the use of reflexivity and that the relationships in the research findings have taken into consideration the circumstances of the research act.

The author kept a reflective journal in which she explored her ideas, feelings and issues. This process was used both for consciousness raising and for exploring feelings about issues encountered. By providing a picture in the journal of the impressions gained during the visits the author found that the immediacy of the impressions returned and through exploration was strengthened. Box 1.2 shows an example of one of these notes.

> ## Box 1.2   Reflexive notes
>
> **Author's reflexivity: thought of getting old**
> My family encouraged me to work on my research but something that I have
> observed today has bothered me and the work was depressing. I imagine how
> difficult it must be for the older frail, but intellectually aware, person and to think about
> getting old. All the things we have to adapt to and tolerate like sharing a room with
> strangers, the food, being in pain or just bored.

Categorising the data – analytic induction

Analytic induction is concerned with presenting statements about regularities and then seeking to verify them using evidence from the empirical data. With analytic induction the author started by inspecting the data and then proceeded to study a section of the data to see whether the latter related to it. The progressive modification is guided by developing theoretical ideas.

The author was concerned with the individual situations of the nurses, the aim being to describe whether a nurse's practice was compatible with propositional theoretical accounts of those situations observed. The writing of memos enabled the author to develop an analytic approach and to be guided by the reflexive ideas and perspectives as described by Hammersley and Atkinson (1995). The author identified the wide variety of literature from nursing journals, textbooks and internet database searches that could be used by the nurses in older people's nursing in their practice.

The method used to categorise the data from the non-participant observations and semi-structured interviews in the first stage of the data analysis was based on content analysis (Lincoln and Guba, 1985). The aim was to produce a record of the themes and issues addressed in the observations and interviews within a system of categories. The development of the categories and themes allowed the author to organise the large volume of clinical data. The author continued to write memos during the content analysis, recording ideas and thoughts that occurred as she worked through the data, indicating possible links or gaps between the categories and themes. Through this process the theorising and generating of relationships between the themes began. The aim was for the author to become fully aware of the experiences of the nurses. The transcripts were read through and headings written down to describe aspects of the content.

A computerised method was chosen to store and analyse the data, which was saved as text files; the data was then imported into a database and this validated the information derived from the data. It is widely recognised that nursing knowledge is complex and varied in nature. Johns (1996) has incorporated Carper's framework in the development of a reflective framework. This framework is widely cited in the literature and advocated on nursing studies courses within some British universities (Johns, 1996). It was therefore decided to utilise Carper's taxonomy (Carper, 1978) as a way of analysing the research data in this study, in order to explore the practice theory.

It was hoped that each item of data could be placed in one of the four patterns – art, science, aesthetics and ethical issues – as a means of identifying the sources of knowledge in the data. However, the author found that the data did not always fit into Carper's taxonomy because the categories were inappropriate and had many statements that could not be fitted into the categories at all. The framework did not allow the author to be focused enough on the emerging informal practice theories. It was often difficult to fit in aspects of the clinical nurses' work that referred to the nurses' interactions with patients and the underlying therapeutic nature of that care because the categories were inappropriate for the clinical data. For example, issues relevant to the comfort needs in particular aspects of care, the hopes for the patients' future home care, and the interactions between the colleagues and obvious multidisciplinary collaboration were examples of the discrepancy that existed between the patterns of knowing. All of these involved the nurses' use of self in a meaningful way in their relationships with patients, families and colleagues. Carper's framework was found to be unhelpful and was not used further.

Qualitative analysis continued is an inductive process. The analysis of ethnographic data is not a simple one-off activity, but is continuous throughout the fieldwork stage and the writing-up stage.

Content analysis allowed the author to study the theoretical issues and to gain an understanding of the data. As a research analysis technique, content analysis provides a systematic and objective means to describe and quantify issues that arise. Thus, a detailed process of content analysis of the data was achieved. It also permits greater certainty in data analysis by reducing data into categories. Computerised categorisation and analysis make the process of categorisation systematic and hence rigorous. It was, therefore, a practical method of organising and analysing this qualitative study.

The categories identified in the research were examined under the higher-order headings and it was then possible to reduce the number of categories into themes. Theory was linked to the data as it emerged and became a source of validity (Denzin and Lincoln, 2005).

Comparing the findings with the literature on care of older people

Pause for thought

Do you think that all nursing theory is relevant to your work as a nurse? If not, what sources of theory do you use in your practice?

The author identified the wide variety of literature that nurses in older people's nursing could use in their practice. However, it should be noted that the volume of literature available is unmanageable unless there is a process of selection in the material. The literature available came from many sources including:

- journals
- books
- reports
- theses
- conference proceedings
- circulars
- computer databases.

The author decided to utilise all the current literature in the care of older people available to the nurses. These were:

- textbooks on older people's nursing
- periodicals and journals
- nursing procedure manuals
- nursing policy documents.

The textbooks and journals were an example of nursing literature that contains the most current information and reports in regard to general trends, issues and research; they reflect any contemporary changes in the discipline. These textbooks and journals were limited to literature in the last five years and were limited to older people's nursing practice. All journals were used, including those read by the nurses in this study: primary journals, such as the *Advanced Journal of Nursing*, which publish original research material; and secondary journals, which often contained a brief synopsis of research but were generally written in less technical terms.

Books on older people were also a source of information. A point to consider was whether a book had a single author or multiple authors (in the case of the latter, there is sometimes variation in the quality of individual chapters). Reports in the form of research studies were also used. These had probably reached only a limited audience of nurses since they were not easily accessible; nurses might only use the university library if they were on academic courses at the university.

Theses and dissertations were available but again limited to library use only. However, the university library had access to these through inter-library loans. Government circulars, via the Department of Health, and Clinical Effectiveness bulletins were available in the search; however, the distribution of these documents and access to them was limited for the nurses working with older people.

Internet searches of databases allowed easy access to research sites and electronic journals and also made available a large number of nursing resources, ranging from general topic areas on older people's nursing to more specific subject areas. It was possible to access the most up-to-date information from this source. This system of literature searching was only available to the nurses via the library sources.

In addition, the Cumulative Index for Nursing and Allied Health Literature (CINAHL) was used. Other sources included the British Nursing Index (BNI), PubMed and MEDLINE to identify key texts, and the internet using the search engine Google. All this literature allowed the researcher to make comparisons of the research data with the literature on that topic as an ongoing process during the data collection and data analysis.

Factor isolation

Following the content analysis, a second stage of analysis took place; this was factor isolation, to identify the informal practice theories in use by the nurses. Dickoff and James (1968a) assert that a factor-isolating theory gives a complete set of significant factors or names for these factors for relevant kinds of real situations. Descriptive theories such as factor-isolating theories describe the event, a situation or a relationship, identifying its components, and identifying the circumstances in which it occurs.

Meleis (2006) further offered an approach that is comprehensible and can be applied in factor isolation. There are no recipes for knowledge building and no one particular way of doing it. Descriptive theory building such as factor isolation looks at the factors present and identifies major elements and events. This involved a basic level of conceptualisation, which aimed to classify and label. Meleis (2006) suggests that labelling should occur in knowledge development and that as the process unfolds the label applied in the first instance may change several times. Factor-isolating theory is one that helps to label factors. The significance of this kind of theory is to help in future studies to refer back to those factors that relate to the subject of nursing care of older people.

Without this first-level theory development we have no concepts, and without concepts we have no relationships. Dickoff and James (1968b) have advocated this level of theory development, in which they had engaged even before they published their work on theory development in nursing. Meleis (1995) developed role supplementation and role insufficiency. Despite this, factor isolation is an area in nursing research that has not been well developed.

The author began to explore the themes from the first-stage research data in order that a more precise description of factors could be adopted; this stage was the labelling stage. The purpose of labelling was to develop descriptions of the factors of practice theory identified in the themes. These labels used the language of the nurses as discussed in the research data, because it was felt that it would be more easily understood and conveyed to others.

Factor isolation began with the author working through each theme, reading each word in each theme on the statement. Starting with the first line of the statement, the author explored what factor or label was needed in order to describe or to account for the issues discussed in the statement. The factor 'advising' occurred frequently within the theme of nutrition and was directly related to the nurses giving advice on issues relating to nutrition (see Table 1.1). The author explored the theoretical literature on advising to examine whether this information was the same as, or could be found in, the academic textbook theory.

The process of analysis is a part of the ethnographic research process, and not a stage that begins once the data collection is

Table 1.1   Factor isolation: advising identified as a factor in the theme of nutrition

Statement	ID number
Nasogastric feeding	224
Nurse explains the feeding regime	2224
Talks and explains nutrition	2231
Nurse sits on the bed and explains and encourages fluids	2237
Asks about the home situation and cooking and advises	2237
Understands patient apprehension about nasogastric feeding	2864
Advises nil by mouth to the patient	2868
Asks the son for help with feeding	2869
Fluid balance recording	2911
Advises about problems at home in dietary habits	2073
Identifies husband to help with feeding	2075
Encourages husband to see the dietician	2073
Identifies problems in dietary habits	2073

complete. The method of ethnographic analysis involved a constant process of explaining the actions and interactions discovered through the experiences of the research. Initially, description stays closest to the original data, but selectively organising and focusing on categories and themes or narratives. However, the transformation of data usually goes beyond this descriptive stage, with general inferences made about them.

Subjecting the data to rigorous analysis offers a way to achieve research credibility; it must be noted that it is not possible to generalise from qualitative research. Such analysis moved a bit further from description into somewhat broader interpretation, and the specific nature and strength of the link with the data remained clear. The relatively formal analysis of ethnographic data began with the development of categories and then proceeded to explore relationships. The analysis was then refined, modified, challenged, and sometimes rejected. It required the author to make explicit the theoretical influences that structured the research process as well as the way in which they implicated the research findings.

Denzin and Lincoln (2005) suggest factors are identified and that we should find patterns of these in the data analysis. The tendency to equate meanings or relationships with patterns in the analysis of qualitative data becomes a commitment to the process of looking for resemblances. The analysis of qualitative data could involve searching for resemblances and assigning a label to the data in the belief that doing so is necessary for eventual meaningful interpretation, and looking at possible similarities among specific instances to show a relationship between these.

Hammersley and Atkinson (1995) suggest that researchers examine various empirical instances of the relationship. By following this advice, the author was able to compare actual instances of that relationship between the ideas, and on the basis of these comparisons isolate some of the possible characteristics of their relationship and compare further instances of the relationship in order to develop and refine it. Any explanation for the patterns of human behaviour must trace out the meanings involved and consider how they form part of the interactional context (Hammersley and Atkinson, 1995). This approach was adopted for the final stage of analysis; the purpose of this was to discover the relationship of the factors to each other, and to the context of the practice of older people's nursing.

Relationships in the data

The author was conscious that the major strengths of qualitative research lie in its emphasis upon understanding the subject of interest (Lincoln and Guba 1985; Denzin and Lincoln, 2005), which was informal practice theory. This led to a style of factors relating analysis that sought to study informal practice theory in the context of holistic nursing care of the older people. Qualitative data analysis placed the complexity and individual nature of care of older people at the centre of the identification of the relationships in the analysis. Identifying the relationships within the data demonstrated fully the dynamic nature of the cycle of informal practice theory building within practice situations and was supported by the literature on informal practice theory (Ebbutt, 1985; Elliott, 1991; Schon, 1991; Eraut, 1994). It was inappropriate to test relationships in a cause-and-effect manner as in positivist research, as data stripping would have lost the meaning and context of the research data (Lincoln and Guba, 1985). The task was therefore to discover if there were any relationships between the factors in an interpretive mode of inquiry (Hammersley and Atkinson, 1995; Denzin and Lincoln, 2005) in which, using the author's reflexivity, the author was able to identify the relationships and meanings the factors identified through observation of the nursing of older people.

Conclusion

The analysis of the data will be presented in Part II of the book, which will show the factors of practice theory and a new framework for care of older people. The next chapter looks at the theoretical underpinning of the research: theory development in the practice of nursing. It will explore how nursing knowledge is viewed generally, and what nurses value and use mostly in their nursing practice.

Suggested reading

Finlay, L. and Gough, B. (2003) *Reflexivity: A Practical Guide for Researchers in Health and Social Sciences* (London: Blackwell Publishing). This book recognises the value of reflexivity to researchers and provides a means to navigate the field. It is a practical guide that explores reflexivity at different stages of the research process.

Jamieson, A. and Victor, C. (2002) *Researching Ageing and Later Life* (London: Open University Press). This edited book addresses the methodological challenges entailed in studying the process of ageing and life course changes, as well as the experience of being old. The book focuses on the theory and practice of doing research using a wide range of examples and case studies.

Polit, D. and Beck, C. (2004) *Nursing Research Principles and Methods*, 7th edition (London: Lippincott Williams and Wilkins). This edition has made research awareness relevant in an environment that is increasingly focused on evidence-based practice.

Chapter 2

Theory development in nursing

This chapter:

identifies what is a nursing theory and how nursing theory is developed;
identifies what are the different levels of nursing theory;
discusses in detail what is practice theory.

The theory of nursing

This chapter looks more closely at the ways and levels in which theory of nursing is viewed and used in nursing practice. It explores some of the key concepts of nursing theory as it is applied to the practice of nursing and will build up a picture of the complex processes that underpin practice and theory.

Nurses in practice are able to utilise knowledge from a wide variety of sources and, because of this, there has been an urgency for nursing to develop research-based knowledge for practice. Nursing research focuses primarily on developing knowledge about nursing and its practice, including the care of persons in health and illness. Despite this research activity there are suggestions in the nursing literature that the divide between theory and practice has been growing. There is a belief also that many of the nursing theories are irrelevant to trained nurses (Benner, 1984). This may have contributed to a dissonance between 'what and how nurses know' and 'what and how nurses do'. There is increasing concern about the theory and practice gap in clinical practice, practitioners having to rely on their intuition and experience since traditional scientific knowledge often does not fit the uniqueness of the situation.

Why research practice theory?

The author's initial interest in the issue of practice theory arose from her work as a nurse lecturer in teaching nursing theory – and in particular reflective practice – to students on graduate study courses within a British university. During these courses, nurses were encouraged through reflective practice sessions in experiential workshops to reflect on incidents from their own practice. During the course the critical incident analysis was developed using reflective frameworks (Carper, 1978; Meizirow, 1990; Johns, 1996) to explore the nurses' knowledge that underpinned their practice.

It seems that reflective practice has gained interest within nurse education and practice, its purpose being to enable practitioners to assess, understand and learn through their lived experience and from this to develop an awareness and increased effectiveness within their own nursing practice. Reflective practice is seen as a model for structured reflection on experience. Within this process any discrepancies between desirable practice and actual practice are made visible and become the focus of discussion and analysis in tutorial sessions. Essentially, learning in this way is by a process of enlightenment, empowerment and emancipation (Johns, 1996): 'enlightenment', to understand who one is in the context of nursing practice; 'empowerment', to take action and make changes in one's own practice; and 'emancipation', to be liberated from previous ways of working so as to become more clinically effective.

It became evident to the author in these reflective practice sessions that the knowledge from the nurses' critical incidents was not as readily available, or the same, as that found in the nursing textbooks or the nursing literature. The work of Argyris and Schon (1974) has been increasingly pertinent to nurse teachers involved in teaching reflective practice. Through exposure to this work the author became interested in the issue of practice theory, in terms of what nursing knowledge is used by nurses in practice. The main issues that the author identified were:

> There has not been, to date, any tradition in the United Kingdom of research into the practice theory nurses use within the discipline itself.
> Practice theory frequently involves what might be termed 'tacit knowledge' (Polanyi, 1967) and as such it is difficult to define. When nurses are asked to describe what it is they know, they find

it difficult to articulate this and often provide descriptions that are superficial or inappropriate to their practice.

Practice theory remains essentially concealed in action and does not become legitimised as nursing knowledge and theory because it has not been subject to research methods and therefore does not become published.

Benner (1984) suggested that theory to guide practice is embedded in practice itself. Theory and practice are as important as each other. However, clinical situations are always more varied and complicated than theoretical accounts; therefore clinical practice should be explored for further research enquiry and knowledge development. Thus questions arise about the usefulness to nurses in the clinical situation of the theory and knowledge that has been written in textbooks or developed through scientific research, and whether this type of knowledge is the same as that which underpins practice. Moreover, Benner's (1994) findings are significant to nursing in that practice theory remains as nurses' experiences and does not become legitimised as nursing theory because practice theory has not been validated by research methods. If this is the case, there is a wealth of knowledge that has never been captured and that disappears as each generation of nurses leaves the profession. However, an important issue for consideration was, 'What is meant by practice theory?' and 'Who should decide the relevance of knowledge that is useful in nursing practice?' The following sections will review levels of nursing theories available to nurses.

Grand theories of nursing

It appears that many authors have believed that there is value in the application of nursing theory to the discipline of nursing. However, many nursing theories seem to be abstract and nurses in practice find them difficult to understand or use (Meleis, 2006). In many ways, nursing theory and research have not influenced practice as much as was expected to be the case. In addition, there is evidence to suggest that nurses in the clinical situation question the usefulness of abstract grand theories and consider that their use is limited in the practice of patient care.

One way of viewing theory refers to the actual products of theoretical enquiries, presented in the form of general principles, laws and explanations. Alternatively, formal theory can refer to the framework of thoughts that structures and guides theoretical activity. Despite this, there has been a tremendous amount of effort within the discipline of nursing to generate formal grand theories.

Nursing theorists have been developing grand nursing theories in the tradition of classical seventeenth-century science, involving an atomistic, mechanistic view of the person. In addition to being mechanistic, nursing theories have been viewed as having superior status over nursing practice. This formal knowledge in nursing has been viewed as a product to be used, and the role of the nurse in practice developing knowledge has been overlooked.

Many of the nursing traditional definitions (Rogers, 1970; King 1981; Roy, 1984; Leininger 1991; Orem, 2001) were influenced by the logical positivistic received view and appear to dominate most of the formal theories developed in nursing. This perspective is based on the assumption that only a singular reality exists which is universally constructed and objectively measured. Logical positivism strives to prove a cause-and-effect relationship for human experiences (Lincoln and Guba, 1985). Science and theory development based on positivist rationale is considered value free, reducible and isolatable, with knowledge being characterised by identifiable and law-like properties. These properties are used to explain complexities. The logical positivist perspective has influenced formal definitions of nursing theory. It would seem, however, that there has been a disagreement over the definitions of a nursing theory (Table 2.1).

Table 2.1 Definitions of nursing theory

Nursing theory	Definition
McKay (1969)	'logically interrelated sets of confirmed hypotheses' (p. 394)
Dickoff and James (1968a)	'A conceptual system or framework invented for some purpose' (p. 515)
Webster et al. (1981)	'A relationship between events and a set of statements and additionally it advocates that the theory must be formalised' (p. 23)
Meleis (1997)	'A conceptualisation of events and relationships in, or pertaining to, nursing for the purpose of describing, explaining, predicting and prescribing nursing care' (p. 97)

The nature of nursing focuses on persons within the context of their environment, as discussed in the nature of contemporary nursing. Traditional formal theories have insisted on separating the person from the environment. Traditional grand formal nursing theories have attempted to control, predict and explain what nurses are doing, and how patients should be responding. Consequently, nursing has attempted to generate theories from a singular objective reality. However, nursing practice is about complex human responses.

Technical rationality

Technical rationality has been seen as the objective truth, which reflects a view that sees a relationship between formal nursing theories and practice as theory preceding practice. Nursing theorists have developed nursing concepts and models which are abstract and highly theoretical and based on a mechanistic way of approaching nursing care. However, this development of nursing theory has become inconsistent with the practice of nursing and there has been considerable debate in the educational literature regarding the theory and practice gap. Therefore, it is important to consider these developments in education and their relevance to the practice of nursing. The relationship between theory and practice has received much attention in the general educational literature (Schon, 1990; Elliott, 1991; Eraut, 1994; Usher, et al. 1997). In education, for example, there is an ever-increasing body of theoretical literature regarding issues about the logical relationship between theoretical statements and practice. Despite attempts to explain how theory should relate to practice in education, teachers say that formal theory has nothing to do with their everyday problems.

The kind of educational theory through technical rationality that exists is abstract and highly general and such theory does not have any practical purpose for teachers. In the main, the gaps between theory and practice seem to be so incompatible that the entire conceptual framework underlying conventional scientific methods of developing theory is called into question.

Usher et al. (1997) suggest that the technical rational model of scientific rationale assumes that theoretical knowledge must be the foundation of practice because it is research generated, systematic and scientific. Scientific knowledge is seen as having power to make predictions about events and thus can be seen to be able to control situations. The way that technical rationality constitutes the relationship between theory and practice is strongly contested by Usher et al. (1997), based on the premise that theoretical knowledge is neither situational nor action orientated.

Schon (1991) referred to positivism as the technical rational model, as 'the positivist epistemology of practice'. It is a method that has been used in the natural sciences, where research-based evidence is seen as the ultimate form of knowledge. The theory and practice gap is non-existent in the hard sciences because the positivist quantitative approach determines its conduct. Schon (1990) believes that technical rationality, which has been the dominant epistemology of practice based on positivism, has most powerfully shaped professional thinking and the relationship of research, education and practice. He suggests that the practice of rigorous technical problem solving based on scientific knowledge has led to a hierarchical model of professional knowledge that separates theory from practice. This separation has led to a theory–practice gap, with practitioners relying on their intuitive practice derived from their past experiences of similar situations, where technical knowledge does not appear to be appropriate or to fit the uniqueness of the individual situation. The problems faced by practitioners do not appear as singular concepts or as well-formed structures.

The traditional scientific approach to research has its underpinnings in the philosophical paradigm known as positivism. Traditionally, technical rationality as a way of generating knowledge is viewed from the scientific method (see Figure 2.1). The ground of positivist science lies in a theory of knowledge and realist ontology.

Knowledge, according to the realist assumptions, must be attained by an objective reality. The most important characteristic of positivism can be called facts (Silverman, 2006). Positivists believe in the notion of cause and effect and look for explanations in empirical data. The aim of science is to produce a body of knowledge that can enhance our understanding of events and where possible predict, prevent, maintain or change them. The empirical view is regarded as an exact and rational activity. Based on the strength of data collected, empirical rules are arrived at through induction and generalisation. The theory is a form of logical arrangement of empirical rules. The positivist tradition in scientific methodology has been based upon the principle of particular instances of patterns. Laws are treated as certain generalisations of descriptions of these patterns. In turn, theories are reduced to a logical sequence. For the positivist, two

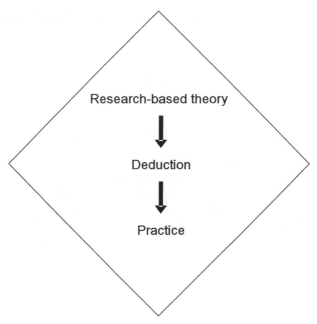

Figure 2.1   The technical rationality model and its relationship between theory and practice

processes govern the task of understanding a formal theory: firstly, the analysis of theoretical discourse, which is aimed at outlining its logical structure; secondly, the revelation of the empirical content of the theory, achieved by identifying those logical consequences of the set of laws which describes the issues.

Levels of nursing theory

Formal grand nursing theory could have been given greater status than practice and used as a universal model of knowledge (Meleis, 2006). In addition to the dispute about definitions of formal nursing theory and the value of nursing theory in practice, there is also a disagreement over types and levels of theory.

Classic theorists Dickoff and James (1968a) cited four levels of theory: meta theory, grand theory, middle-range theory and practice theory. There have been debates over the levels of theory from grand, middle-range and practice theory and the relative contribution of these to nursing knowledge (Meleis, 2006).

Grand theories of nursing are abstract and have been proposed to give some broad perspective to the goals and structures of nursing practice. Some examples of grand theories are nursing models such as Peplau's (1988) exposition of nursing, and its educative function with patients. Subsequent grand theories shifted from a focus on the nurse and patient relationship to a more conceptualised analysis. Rogers (1970) stressed a holistic approach based on the life process of man. A multi-level systems model developed by King (1981) included the major concepts of perception, interpersonal relationships, social systems and health. Johnson (1980) constructed a model of the client as a behaviour system composed of sub-systems. Grand theories have attempted to capture the phenomenological aspects of nursing. Watson (1988) adopted a phenomenological existential orientation in her theory of human care. Others, such as Leininger's (1985) 'Transcultural Care Theory' (see Leininger, 1991), considered cultural factors. Grand theories were thought to provide global perspectives for nursing practice education and research, which could be used by nurses in practice. However, there have been criticisms that these theories are limited, as they presently exist. It seems that by virtue of their generality and abstractness many grand theories represent a theoretical interpretation of what nursing should be, but nurses in practice do not find them useful. Nursing as an emerging profession has been faced with the problem of describing and defining nursing; the development of nursing models is seen as a way of describing nursing more clearly (Meleis, 2006).

Reed and Robbins (1991) suggested that nursing models and grand theory perspectives are difficult to apply in an individual nursing situation because practice is more complex than theoretical accounts allow. Without doubt, nurses do appear to struggle to relate to the assumptions that underpin the model of nursing. A number of authors have identified the increasing amount of literature describing grand nursing theory (Walker and Avant, 1994; Meleis, 2006). There is also a suggestion that the use of such theory will offer benefits in patient care. However, despite this encouragement to use formal nursing theory there is growing discontent since the academic theory has seemingly failed in practice. The formal nursing theories cited are abstract theoretical accounts and do not appear to be consistent with practice. Whilst these ideas are being generated, there is also the view that nursing should develop a unique body of knowledge that it can call its own and recognise the practice element of nursing care (Meleis, 2006). Some critics believe that such an aim is not possible. Other authors suggest that the development of middle-range theories should become more focused on patient problems and develop a theory of nursing in doing so (Davies and Nolan, 2006; McCormack and McCance, 2006). However, there has been a shift from grand theories to middle-range theories to develop a formal theory of nursing.

Pause for thought

Reflect on the use of nursing models in your daily practice.

Middle-range theories

An alternative view that has been suggested to develop practice is that nurses should develop middle-range theories that consider a smaller range of variables. Davies (2005) suggests that mid-range nursing theories are useful tools in helping to understand the scope of nursing practice in a range of contexts and situations. Meleis's theory of nursing transitions and relatives' experiences of nursing-home entry provides a mid-range theory of nursing. Meleis provided findings from a constructivist study of relatives' experience of nursing-home entry. Data from the study generated 37 interviews involving 48 close family members of older people who had recently moved to a nursing home. The mid-range theory of nursing transitions shows how nurses are able to use such information for supporting relatives throughout the period of the older person's move to a nursing home.

What is practice theory?

It seems that the problem of formal nursing theories not representing practice could be resolved by acknowledging the importance of individuality and subjectivity of the nurse–patient interaction in the development of theory. The development of formal theory in nursing has denied research being developed from practice and could well be the answer to the development of nursing theory. Benner and Wrubel (1989) advised that theory building in nursing must be informed by real-world experience and then be subjected to theoretical interpretation. Benner suggested that formal theories of nursing have not been shaped by the practice of nurses, and she states: 'A theory is needed that describes, interprets and explains not an imagined ideal of nursing but actual expert nursing as it is practised day to day' (p. 5). Nurses appear to have struggled to adapt care to theoretical frameworks rather than from nursing care itself.

However, Schon (1990) reminds us that the nature of professional work is exceedingly complex and often fast moving, with decisions being made by the nurse about the best alternatives there and then. He further suggests that different professions share common characteristics:

> Professionals face complex problems in their day-to-day work. There are often no definitely right or wrong answers, but only good and not so good ones.
> When making decisions, professionals draw on a knowledge base, which is broad, deep and multifaceted.
> The context in which professionals use their knowledge and skills is very important.
> Professional knowledge is not just about having expert skills.
> It is often difficult for professionals to say or write about what it is they know and how they use their knowledge. (Schon, 1990: 9)

Professional knowledge involves much more than simply applying the body of knowledge; it also requires the cognitive skills to use that knowledge critically and creatively. It is this practice knowledge generated by practitioners in action that writers such as Schon (1991) Benner (1984) and Davies and Nolan (2006) believe needs to be explored to provide a body of knowledge that is directly relevant to the realities of practice.

In order to become more focused on the theory on which nurses base their practice, Morse (1995) suggests a qualitative framework that uses actual clinical data to develop concepts of nursing, and suggests an inductive approach to theory building and concept development (which was the approach taken in the study discussed in this book). Such an inductive approach would not seek to test hypotheses but rather to describe and explain the world of nursing.

Despite these complications, Benner (1984) claimed that practice theory has been seen to have benefits for nursing practice and the development of nursing knowledge. It seems then that professional nursing involves much more than applying the body of knowledge; it also requires the ability to apply that knowledge in patient care. This may require the nurse to use their self-awareness and to learn from their experience. It is this professional knowledge, generated by nurses in action, that needs to be further explored in order to develop an understanding about the knowledge that is directly related to patient care.

Benner (1984) focused on the proposition that perceptual awareness is central to good nursing judgement and contends that practice knowledge accrues over time. Benner's research explored nurses' discretionary judgement used in clinical situations. The central premise of Benner's work was that 'expertise develops when the clinician tests and refines propositions, hypotheses and principle based expectations in actual practice situations' (p. 3). It seems from Benner's account that nurses are able to achieve personal knowledge by drawing on past experiences in similar situations in the present. Benner argued that each expert nurse has his or her own repertoire of paradigm cases that is unique to them: a collection of personal knowing that is different from formal theory. Benner discussed the notion of expertise in clinical practice, but did not seem to explore the ways that nurses formulated and tested hypotheses in action.

Benner identified six areas of practical knowledge that she claims can be observed in nursing experts. Research is needed to make clinical know-how public so that it can be extended and refined. Benner suggested that each area could be explored using ethnographic and interpretative strategies to identify and extend practical knowledge. The six areas are:

1. Graded qualitative distinctions, which can be elaborated and refined as nurses compare their judgements in actual patient care situations.
2. Common meanings, which are developed by nurses working with common ideas. Meanings are developed over time and shared.
3. Assumptions, expectations and sets, which relate to practical situations in which nurses learn to expect a certain course of events.
4. Paradigm cases and personal knowledge in particular situations that stand out in nurses' minds and could alter their actions in the future.
5. Maxims, which are cryptic comments that only make sense if there is already a deep understanding of the situation.
6. Unplanned practices, which are activities that nurses may have had delegated to them. They have taken them on because they

are constantly at the bedside and because of this have become highly skilled in these practices. (Benner, 1984: 54)

Benner followed the philosopher Ryle (1949) who referred to knowledge as 'know how' and 'know that' knowledge. 'Knowing how' consists of practical skills, sometimes described as the art of nursing. However, 'know that' knowledge consists of propositional knowledge found in textbooks and includes formal statements. Benner claimed that experienced nurses are unable to articulate all they know and said that their knowledge is qualitatively different from that of beginners. Benner (1984) suggests there are situations where the nurse draws on his or her experiences, selects an appropriate action and finds a way of synthesising this information so that it can be applied to a similar situation. She explored the practice of 'expert nurses' and suggested that experts view the situation holistically; she found that much of their knowledge is embedded in practice and displayed by competent practitioners in practice situations. Expertise in nursing exists when the nurse has developed the ability to use appropriate nursing knowledge and skilled judgements in delivering patient care. Such ability requires that the expert nurse has abstract knowledge but has developed the intellectual capacity to contextualise and to adjust this knowledge in particular cases.

If Benner's propositions of the stages of expert knowledge are accurate it could be possible for some practitioners who have not reached the level of expertise based on their experience to have one type of knowledge but not the other. A student nurse in their first year of training might have textbook knowledge or information but not the practice knowledge in that subject. However, the expert nurse should have both – a combination of 'knowing how' and 'knowing that' – and it is the development of the experiential 'know how' knowledge that develops expertise. However, Benner pointed out that experience does not simply refer to working in an area in nursing over a period of time, and that there is a difference between the competent level and the proficient and expert levels. According to Benner, expertise is concerned with developing intuitively and responding to practice situations from a body of personal tacit knowledge, a collection of past paradigm cases. It could be the case that the difference between novice and expert is the degree to which parts of the activity have been 'chunked'. In nursing the 'chunks' are the activities that nurses learn such as procedures and principles of nursing care, initially in a theoretical way. Applied to the practice situation, these chunks may be groups of past paradigm cases as identified by Benner. Therefore the difference between the expert and the novice is the degree to which the nursing activities are chunked together hierarchically.

Concerns are expressed by Benner and other theorists (Rolfe et al., 2001) about the shortcomings of the positivist scientific approach to theory development in nursing. Benner suggested that what appears to be missing from positivist scientific approaches to theory development is a direct link to nursing practice to generate the informal theory of nursing from practice itself. An approach that provides a link with practice could provide opportunities to develop knowledge that has meaning for nurses in practice.

Carper's (1978) seminal paper analysing ways of knowing in nursing has been a well-referenced paper in the nursing literature. Carper suggested that the body of knowledge which serves as the basis for nursing practice has patterns, which she has labelled empirics, aesthetics, ethics and personal knowing. These patterns may serve as a yardstick for what may be expected and detail ways of thinking about the complex and varied nature of nursing.

Empirical knowledge can be seen as providing a scientific research base to nursing. This is gained through systematic investigation, observation and testing and is embedded within the positivist paradigm. Aesthetic knowledge is concerned with the actions of nursing. This type of knowledge involves perception, understanding and empathy and acknowledges the value of everyday experiences of practitioners; it can also be linked to actions described as intuitive.

With personal knowledge the nurse approaches the patient with a view to establishing a therapeutic relationship. The patient is a person with his or her own beliefs and values in the creation of self. It was Menzies (1960) who reported that nurses sometimes distance and detach themselves as a defence against anxiety caused by personal giving of oneself. Ethical patterns of knowing require an understanding of different philosophical positions, as to what is good or should be desired, and what is right. This essentially enables the nurse to deal with complex moral judgements and have greater awareness about what is involved in making moral choices and being responsible for the outcome.

Informal practice theory

There have been suggestions of how the theory and practice gap can be closed by a model of praxis. These ideas originated in the work of Stenhouse (1975) and Hammersley and Atkinson (1995), the key instigators of the debate about researchers and practitioners in teacher education. Stenhouse claimed that professional development of teachers' knowledge depended on their capacity to adopt a research stance. Stenhouse advocated that teachers adopt a research model to underpin their teaching, which should include teachers producing accounts of their reflections on their own experiences. Stenhouse suggested that action research with the aim of reflection in and on practice develops an improvement in a given practice situation through a search for explanation. A number of experiential learning models have arisen from studies of learning in practice. They are important to consider because they have gained prominence in education and practice. In the educational literature there are theories of experiential learning (Lewin, 1958; Argyris and Schon, 1974; Kolb, 1985). Common to all is the centrality of experience at the source of learning. Lewin's model of action research is described as a problem-solving approach.

Carr and Kemmis (2002) discuss views about how formal theory is developed and the belief that problems in education can only be solved by experimental methods of science, that is, through technical rationality. The central point in the issue is that there has been dispute and a more general conflict between positivist and interpretative approaches to social enquiry. Carr and Kemmis discuss the notion of theory. They suggest that all theories are the product of some practical activity and that all practical activities are guided by theory. They say that a practice is not a thoughtless behaviour that exists separately from theory and to which theory can be applied. In addition, all practices have theory embedded in them and it is just as true for the practice of theoretical pursuits as it is for those practical activities such as teaching or nursing. Carr and Kemmis make the point that the twin assumptions that all theory is non-practical and all practice is non-theoretical are misguided; and that the interpretative approach which rejects the idea of the practitioner as a user of scientific theories but recognises practitioners' research should be recognised as being part of the theories that practitioners have themselves acquired through their experiences. The point that Carr and Kemmis are making is that practitioners cannot depend on methods of scientific theories but instead must use methods for uncovering the theories in their own experiences. It is the connection between the theoretical accounts produced through research and the practitioners' own theorising that needs to be made clearer.

Carr and Kemmis (2002) suggest that there is a basic understanding that knowledge can be developed in three different ways: firstly, through logical argument, as in philosophy; secondly, through empirics; and lastly, through pragmatics, which is to say that we know something that in our experience works for us. Practitioners' knowledge is legitimised by pragmatism and refers to their practical wisdom. If an action is successful for the practitioner they will repeat it until such time as it no longer works.

Practical wisdom

Practical wisdom is not about scientific knowledge; it is accomplished through an understanding of a particular situation: no two situations are ever the same, they are unique. Elliott (1991) discusses teachers' practical wisdom, which he refers to as the practitioner's capacity to take the right course of action when faced with particular, complex situations. Elliott suggests that the teacher's knowledge is not in theoretical propositions but as a reflectively processed repertoire of cases. Practical knowledge in the context of individual situations cannot be universal or the product of grand theories because it cannot be taken away from the context in which that individual situation occurs, and each individual situation is unique – one of a kind. Elliott referred to practical wisdom or knowledge as knowing how to act in relation to the circumstances of a particular situation or context. This, of course, may allow the practitioner to use general or universal theoretical knowledge. Practical knowledge, in this instance, refers to the fact that contexts are not particular instances of a universal characteristic as they have too many unique and indeterminate features. Elliott advocates practitioner-based research as the way to improve practice, and argued that the validity of such research depends entirely on its 'usefulness in helping people to act more intelligently and skilfully'. Elliot suggested that the researcher should employ her or his own professional judgement in order to decide the usefulness of research for practice. He advocates that single-case research using action research methods can be conducted by experienced practitioners. On discussing issues of validity of such action, research suggests that action research of this kind could provide for naturalistic generalisations or transferability (Lincoln and Guba, 1985). Usher et al. (1997) referred to the knowledge used in practice situations as informal theory. Informal theory generates new theory as it is modified in practice in each individual situation.

Informal theories are not the same as traditional formal theories, which are applied to practice rather than developed from practice. More importantly, Usher et al. (1997) note that in developing and testing informal theory, changes are made in practice itself. Informal theory in practice thus has a direct effect on practice through action. They suggest that a context cannot be acted upon through the application of rules across all contexts. Practical knowledge is not seen as what is right in principle or in theory. In addition, they show why informal theory is not a matter of skills. Whilst it is 'know how', it is not the 'know how' of techniques. Informal theory is about being in a situation, whether it is as teacher, nurse or practitioner. Finding oneself in the circumstance of having to do something that is the right and appropriate response for that situation, the practitioner must draw on their own resources, which may be propositional theory or the practitioner's own informal theory or an applied combination of both. Usher and colleagues suggest that reflection in action takes place in action in real-life situations.

Usher et al. (1997) identify that the relationship between informal theory and practice is different from the relationship between formal propositional theory and practice. Propositional theory informs practice in a somewhat prescriptive way, seen in healthcare in terms of protocols, guidelines and standard care plans, for example. Informal theory and practice are seen as mutually dependent and follow a cycle where practice produces theory; theory modifies practice, which generates new theory, as seen in Figure 2.2, from Rolfe (1999).

The importance of informal theory is that the practitioner is able to solve problems in practice, through a process of testing, modifying, re-testing and experimenting, there and then in practice. Formal propositional theory, as discussed earlier in grand nursing theories, attempts to dictate to practitioners what they should do in a given situation in a causal way.

Carr (1986) discussed the practitioner's ability to research his or her own informal theory in practice by action research. Here the practitioner develops a deep subjective relationship to describe the situation as he or she experiences it. Single-case research is established in

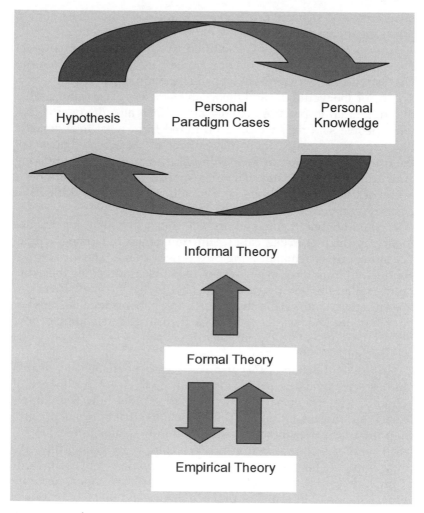

Figure 2.2   Reflexive practice in action. Reprinted from Rolfe (1999), with permission from Elsevier.

other disciplines such as sociology through ethnographic studies (Hammersley and Atkinson, 1995).

Reflection

Elliott (1991) made the point that the researcher should employ his or her own professional judgement in the case of the researcher being the experienced practitioner. Elliot saw the main aim of practitioner-based research as the improvement of practice.

Argyris and Schon (1974) identified two levels of informal practice theories: theories of action or espoused theories, and theories in use. Espoused theory refers to what an individual, when questioned, says he or she would do, and theory in use refers to explaining what the individual in practice actually does. They also discovered that what people said they would do differed from what they actually did. Espoused theories, then, may be seen as the accepted norms of the nursing profession or propositional theory about what nursing and nurses ought to do. Theories in use are the practitioner's responses to the particulars of a situation, which are difficult to describe, but observed in the nurse's behaviour.

It could be that 'theories in use' are thus a synonym for practice theory, as 'theories in use' capture the uniqueness of nursing in practice situations as actual nursing care is performed. 'Theories in use' are derived from the perspectives of the nurse undergoing the experience, rather than from a discussion about what we might do or did in a situation. If nursing is about nurturing patients to make sense of our situations and health experiences, then an understanding of how nurses develop and utilise our 'theories in action' is vital knowledge for nursing.

Argyris and Schon (1974) also conducted a number of research studies across various professional groups to develop a theory of competent interpersonal practice and to explore how individuals learn in the practice situation. They concluded that informal practice theories, or theories in action, underpin human action. 'We cannot learn what someone's theory in use is simply by asking him. We must construct his theory in use from observation of his behaviour of practice' (p. 24). They believe theories in use are a more accurate representation of informal or practice theory and that a practitioner may not always be aware that he or she possesses certain action theories. These informal and practice theories include values, strategies and assumptions that inform individual patterns of interpersonal behaviour. However, Schon conducted research through observation of practitioners' behaviour and suggested that it is possible to explore the theories in action. An informal practice theory, therefore, can be a proposition that states practice; it guides not only practice but also the way the practitioner interacts with others. In nursing there are situations where the nurse draws on his or her experience and selects an appropriate action to find a way of synthesising the practice theory, and will apply it again when the situation is similar. The development of nursing praxis and the dynamic nature in which informal theories are constructed is crucial to the development and understanding of the nature of nursing; it should be an important area for exploratory nursing research to add to the body of knowledge about informal theory in practice.

Pause for thought

Have you ever been in a position where your own responses in a nursing situation have been difficult to describe to others?

Practice theories can thus be seen as 'theories in use', which capture the uniqueness of nursing in practice situations as actual nursing care is performed. 'Theories in action', which produce informal practice theories, are from the perspectives of the nurse undergoing the experience, rather than from an abstract discussion about what they might do or did in a situation. Acknowledging that informal theories are different in their construction from traditional formal theories applied to practice, which are constructed from practice, is an extremely important issue when debating the development of the knowledge base for nursing.

Reflection in and on action

Reflection is at the centre of prominent theories of experiential learning (e.g. Boud et al., 1985; Argyris and Schon, 1974). For Boud et al., experience is the starting point and the object of reflection. For Argyris and Schon, experience is the source and testing ground of theories of action that are formulated during reflection in action. Meizirow considers experience to be the ground for transformative learning.

Schon (1991) discusses informal theory and talks of reflection in action which takes place in the practice situation. Practitioners use their personal knowledge to form an informal theory about the practice situation there and then. The practitioners will hypothesise about the possible outcomes of different possible actions that they may use. The practitioner will then apply that experience and reflect on the outcome. This modification happens in action in a reflective cycle as proposed by Schon, seen in Figure 2.3.

Reflection in action occurs during practice when practitioners use

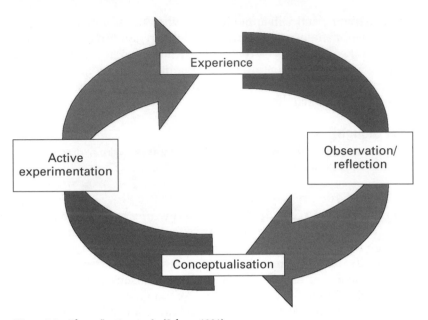

Figure 2.3   The reflective cycle (Schon, 1991)

learning from previous similar experiences and apply it to their current situation. As practitioners, we are using knowledge we have gained from past experiences, which may be tacit knowledge, so that we as practitioners cannot easily discuss what we know. Tacit knowledge is linked to the nature of knowledge by the question 'How do we know what we know?' Tacit knowing is the kind of knowledge in use when we know something only by relying on our awareness of it. Polanyi (1967: 24) defines tacit knowledge as 'knowing more than we can say or articulate'. Polanyi uses the terms 'proximal and distal knowledge' and gives examples based on psychomotor skills, such as the co-ordination of respiration or the action of hammering a nail. Not only is the skilled practitioner unable to describe these skills, but attention to the parts makes the individual unable to perform the whole. Meerabeau (1992) considered the implications of tacit knowledge in a study which acknowledged the existence of tacit knowledge in nursing.

Dickoff and James (1968a) urge that there is a need for researchers who care about the problems of nursing and who see the potential of practice theories to help towards the development of a theory for nursing. Dickoff and James suggest that practice theory describes events, situations or relationships by identifying their properties and goals. Although descriptive theories can have an element of prediction, their contribution to knowledge development is to develop observations and the meanings of those observations regarding nursing. Dickoff and James (1968a) identified practice theory as factor isolating, which is the most basic kind of descriptive theory. Factors are isolated and given names that provide a meaning in abstract terms. The naming process is the first stage in developing factor isolation. Factor-isolating studies utilise normal description, the naming theory being presented in the form of formal concepts with formal definitions. Thus, factor searching or naming studies are descriptive in nature and occur at the exploratory stage of theory development.

Factor-relating practice theories develop categories to further identify their focus. This type of research is descriptive or interpretive and is designed to discover relationships between identified factors and other variables. Jacox (1974) has defined practice theory as 'theory that says given this nursing goal this is the action that the nurse must take to meet the goal'. It is usually a level of nursing theory so basic that it is often overlooked by nurses, and nurses may fail to acknowledge and support the first level of theory development, which is practice theory. Practice theories are those which arise from nursing care, and their purpose is to explain and direct practice. This provides a guide for the evaluation of theories in nursing by legitimising the use of theory in practice and research. Jacox (1974) advises that practice theories are descriptive theories that describe a phenomenon, an event, a situation or a relationship by identifying its properties and its components in some of the circumstances under which it occurs. Although descriptive theories can have an element of prediction, their contribution to knowledge development is to develop observations and the meanings of those observations regarding the phenomena. Practice theory, as factor isolating, is the most basic kind of descriptive theory. Factors are isolated and given names that provide a meaning in abstract terms. The naming process is the first stage in developing factor isolation. Factor-isolating studies utilise normal description, the naming theory being presented in the form of formal concepts with formal definitions. Thus, factor searching or naming studies are descriptive in nature and occur at the exploratory stage of theory development. Factor-relating practice theories develop categories to further identify their focus. I suggest that in an informal theory situation we might question whether or not it is possible to rely on a prescriptive theory as a rigid check-list. In an informal theory, as discussed by Usher et al. (1997), the question arises whether or not a nursing situation has been shaped by the academic theory or whether an informal nurses' theory in action is a feature of the contextualised nature of nursing. This issue is of crucial importance in terms of whether the contextual feature of nursing in human inquiry means that it cannot be possible to know in advance whether a prescriptive theory (textbook) will be success-ful in a particular patient scenario. This point makes a useful ques-tion on which to base research relating to informal practice theory. It was this question that prompted the author to look further into practice-based theory.

Nursing as a practice

Nurses are being challenged to explain the nature of nursing and demands have been made to demonstrate the clinical effectiveness of nursing interventions. And because of the emphasis on clinical effectiveness, nursing has been under increasing pressure to explain what nurses do, suggesting that nursing is no more than clinical interventions that can be measured for clinical and cost effective-ness. This could be to the detriment of nursing as a practice and shows a lack of awareness from policy makers and managers and no real understanding of what the nature of nursing constitutes.

Nursing as a practice does not constitute merely the performing of technical interventions, and nursing is seen to be more than the sum of its parts, although clinical interventions are an aspect of a nurse's work. However, nursing is about preserving, nurturing and protecting and these are the ingredients of nursing care as a practice. These features of nursing are the fundamental aspects of nursing care; they require an investment in another person's wellbeing that gives the patient the strength or will to want to improve. It is these essential elements of nursing that constitute the nature of nursing. If nursing were to be reduced to procedural tasks and administered by unqualified staff then the patient would not be nursed.

To 'nurse' is a process of nourishing, of promoting the develop-ment or progress of something. The meaning also derives from syn-onyms of 'nurse' meaning to heal, to foster and sustain. These descriptions signify that nursing involves a process that is develop-mental, progressive and sustaining, through which wellbeing occurs. This suggests that the nature of nursing is distinguished from other human processes by the characteristics of complexity, integration and wellbeing. The complexity of nursing refers to the number of different types of variables that can be identified in a given situation. It is possible to say that a certain level of complexity is needed for integration to occur. That is when meanings are constructed or identify a pattern in the events experienced. Changes in complexity and integration can be used to explain the nature of healing and the nurse's role in fostering wellbeing in practice.

The meaning of nursing practice seems to resemble and relate to concerns of nurturance, taking charge of, looking after, sustenance, preservation and protection. Nursing practice is about nurses having a genuine interest in helping patients to improve and get better. Nurses recognise what is happening to each patient in complex and difficult situations. They use their ability to reflect in action, which requires on their part a breadth and depth of individual practice knowledge using their experiences of healthcare needs of people. The literature on nursing theory seems to provide accounts of the person in an environment in relation to self-care, stress adaptation, health beliefs and so on, but does not relate to what nursing practice constitutes.

Nursing has been developing a focus on the individual patient and the holistic care of the person. However, new nursing seems in some way to have been hampered and not allowed to flourish by the ethos within the National Health Service that emphasises being cost- and clinically effective. The stress on cost effectiveness may have undermined the practice of nursing. But the insistence that nurses measure the tasks and interventions ignores the very essence of the practice of nursing as nurturing, protecting, holistic, individual care, which is seen to be of low status compared to technical procedures.

Nursing is not about technical skills, but about the motivation and intention on the part of the expert nurse to help the patient to want to get better. It is also clear that nurses' practice is action based. Nursing is viewed as a helping process with the primary focus on interpersonal interactions between the nurse and the patient. The interpersonal nature of nursing provides an important focus for deciding what kind of knowledge and theory is needed in nursing practice.

Sources of knowledge in nursing

Traditional nursing was focused on a medical model of care, which has emphasised a reductionist and biomedical approach to practice.

Many nursing theorists have given traditional definitions of what nursing involves which appear to represent the scientific, technical-rational ways of viewing knowledge and theory building.

Nightingale (1986: 10) contended that to nurse meant having charge of the personal health of a patient, the role of the nurse being seen as 'placing the patient in the best condition for nature to act upon him'. To nurse, then, is to nourish, to look after carefully, and to promote growth and development in the patient.

It is important to examine the nature of nursing knowledge in order to analyse the kinds of knowledge available to enable nurses to practise safely and effectively. Indeed, in order to explain the role of nurses and to understand the complexities of nursing practice, we need to have a clear understanding of the knowledge available. All nurses know nursing; however, what they know and how they know may be different because of their unique experiences and also their ability and desire to reflect upon their experience.

Nursing has historically used knowledge from other disciplines to guide its practice (Fawcett, 1984; Meleis, 2006). Since Nightingale first established formal education for nurses in the United Kingdom, it has been evident that nursing needed knowledge to guide practice. This was initiated in the form of procedures and principles, and, in the main, nursing was viewed as a practical discipline. Nightingale (1986) maintained that the knowledge developed and used by nursing must be distinct from medical knowledge. Nightingale's vision of nursing as an art and a science generated an image of nursing as 'doing' and being practical.

Some of the practical work of nursing has been called a ritual. Formal rituals do require a depth of knowledge, concentration and adherence to correct procedures. Rituals exist in most professions and can demonstrate a rich, in-depth understanding of that discipline. Many rituals can only be performed by those in whom the power has been invested, and they often reflect a deep and complex belief system. Rituals in nursing are important not only in passing down knowledge but also for the socialisation and culture in nursing that we learn from our predecessors. They may also have therapeutic value or other kinds of impact on patients. Wolf (1993) discusses the example of a skilful bath. Looking at nursing as it was traditionally practised allows us to re-examine the nature of the therapeutic bath. Rather than being a therapeutic, comforting and satisfying experience for patients, bathing has been labelled ritualistic and a subject of routine negative comments, or indeed classified as social care. Attention to the impression that the bath has on the patient could return bathing to its prior status as a therapeutic nursing activity. In Wolf's words, 'The bath represents part of the essential character of nursing and is rooted in the beliefs, art and science; it is a channel for many other nursing activities and responses, and as such occupies a necessary part of nursing's repertoire and identity' (1993: 141). On the other hand, Walsh and Ford (1990) suggest that the bath is seen as basic nursing care and is often delegated to social care support workers or junior student nurses. The therapeutic effects of bathing for patients fail to be addressed in such an argument and are either taken for granted or not considered. Wolf (1993) stated that 'Few seem interested in objective searching for knowledge on the effects on bathing patients' (p. 141). Wolf goes on to caution against discarding the bath as routine care and suggests that the ritual of bathing is more than a standardised and repetitive series of activities, and states: 'The bath can be viewed as a healing rite with greater healing power' (p. 141).

It seems that throughout the early part of the twentieth century nursing practice was based on traditions of rules and principles that were passed along through apprenticeship forms of education. Much of what evolved as nursing knowledge was wisdom that came from the experiences of nurses. A lack of a tested, comprehensive theory base for nursing led to the borrowing of theoretical assumptions, concepts and research instruments from other disciplines such as anthropology, sociology, psychology and education. In addition, knowledge for clinical practice was derived from the natural sciences, such as chemistry, pharmacology, bacteriology, physiology and medicine. The development of nursing has been influenced by other disciplines such as sociology, psychology, physiology and anatomy. Whilst it is acknowledged that knowledge from these disciplines can and does support the practice of nursing, these do not constitute nursing knowledge.

Evidence-based knowledge

One of the main strategies to facilitate the use of research has been the development, implementation and evaluation of clinical guidelines. Producing evidence from systematic reviews has also contributed to clinical effectiveness. The aim of nursing research was seen to be the generation of knowledge. However, the application of generalisable research is not always suitable in individual nursing situations. This may have led to a theory and practice gap.

There have been considerable discussions in the nursing literature about the gap between theory and practice and what knowledge nurses use to give care. This can be related over time and many theorists have suggested that there is a theory and practice gap within nursing (Polit et al., 2001). The theory and practice gap is one of the most important issues facing nursing; it calls into question all the efforts put in place by nurse academics, researchers and practitioners to ensure that practice is evidence based, and suggests that science or research is seriously limited in that scientific knowledge can give the appearance of providing proven facts with causal relationships. Even more worrying, it seems that through clinical effectiveness (DoH, 2005), health sciences have become trapped within a particular positivist perspective and this has become the only officially recognised way of knowing. This traditional technical view of knowledge, derived from experimental studies, suggests that practice should always be supported by technical theoretical accounts. That is, research evidence is seen as well-founded knowledge in terms of clinical guidelines, protocols and standardised care plans. The suggestion that practice should always be based on formal theory clearly undermines practice as something that is not as rigorous and scientific, and seems to have been the subject of negative comments by supporters of the scientific rationale.

We need to be more understanding of the nature of the relationship between theory and practice and to seek knowledge that is more appropriate to nurses' work. Much of the knowledge of practice is different from formal theory. In these terms, it is not possible to view practice as being theory led and it suggests that there is in fact a relationship between formal theory and practice; there are examples of this in the use of scientific principles within nursing. However, problems seem to have been created by the claims of nursing theorists that formal nursing theories such as models of nursing also qualify as science. What it represents is an inadequate attempt by formal grand theory to represent knowledge of practice, which cannot in fact be represented in that form.

Conclusion

There are tensions that exist in the discipline of nursing in terms of how theory in nursing is developed. There appears to be disagreement in nursing regarding levels and types of formal nursing theory, and whether theory should be generated from the domain of nursing academia by grand theories and middle-range theories, or whether informal practice theory would provide a basis for developing knowledge about nursing. Nursing is seen to be about nurturing and the nurse–patient relationship is a central pivot to the wellbeing of the patient in contemporary nursing. We have seen in this chapter many sources of knowledge that nurses need to practise safely.

The dominant view of knowledge emphasises abstract, general, theoretical knowledge whilst overlooking practical informal theory about particular clinical situations. Educationalists also argue that the relationships between formal theory and practice, and informal theory in practice have been misunderstood (Meleis, 2006). There are those who support a scientific basis for theory generation whilst others suggest an action research approach. A third approach, typified by Benner, Lawler and Rolfe among others, is to gather nurses' accounts of their practice and to observe nurses at work. With this in mind, this book presents real-life situations from nursing older people, and Chapters 3 and 4 will focus on the theory and practice of gerontological nursing.

Suggested reading

Meleis, A. I. (2006) *Theoretical Nursing: Development and Progress*, 4th edition (London: Lippincott Williams and Wilkins). This comprehensive text looks at the development of theory, and at understanding our current progress and goals in nursing theory. It is designed to stimulate thought processes and to analyse nursing ideas.

Watson, J. (2005) *Caring Science as Sacred Science* (Philadelphia: F. A. Davis Company). The text offers a moral and philosophical foundation for all health personnel interested in caring and in gaining knowledge of caring as it relates to nurse education and practice. This is a very comprehensive and thorough approach to nursing theorists and their work. It provides in-depth descriptions and analysis of nursing theories.

Chapter 3

Building professional knowledge in older people's care

This chapter:

discusses the need for person-centred care of older people;
explains traditional nursing care for older people;
explains the importance of developments in older people's nursing.

Nursing older people

There is shift in thinking about services and care for older people, the latest being the development of person-centred care (Davies and Nolan, 2006). But what is person-centred care? Haven't nurses always been person centred? After all, nursing claims to be 'the caring profession'. Person-centredness implies that nurses should treat older people as individuals and enable them to make decisions about their own care, and it appears to be the guiding principle for the nursing of older people.

'Person centred' is a widely used concept in nursing. However, McCormack and McCance (2006) suggest that there is little evidence demonstrating the relationship between person-centred practice in nursing and the resulting outcomes for patients and nurses. In fact, talking about person centredness has become an established approach to the delivery of healthcare, and indeed is advocated as the way forward in policy documents such as the *National Service Framework for Older People* (DoH, 2001).

Emphasis is placed on the promotion of person-centred care, which has become the pivot of good practice. The *National Service Framework for Older People* was published by the Department of Health in 2001, which, for the first time, set national standards of care for older people in the United Kingdom. Two themes govern this report: the promotion of person-centred care and the rooting out of age discrimination in the National Health Service. Thus, older people and their carers should receive services that respect them as individuals, and which are arranged around their needs. More importantly, nurses need to re-examine the contribution they make to care of older people and consider how they can maximise their knowledge and input around carers. McCormack and McCance (2006) advocate the person-centred nursing framework, the principles of which underpin human science principles, including the centrality of human freedom, choice and responsibility, holism, forms of knowledge, and the importance of relationships. McCormack (2004; McCormack and McCance, 2006) suggests that in the field of gerontological nursing person centredness and person-centred practice is a recurring theme in the modern literature. However, McCormack advises that whilst use of the term 'person-centred practice' has become common, there are very few published research studies in the literature on the subject, and suggests there is a need for further research and development to distinguish between person-centred practice and good quality care for older people.

McCormack (2006) published further findings from a study that was developed through an interactive process; the framework was developed for use in the intervention stage of a large quasi-experimental project that focused on measuring the effectiveness of the implementation of person-centred nursing. The process included mapping of original conceptual frameworks against the person-centred nursing literature, and focus groups with practitioners in a person-centred nursing development project. The person-centred nursing framework comprises four constructs: the care environment; looking at the context in which care is delivered; person-centred processes, which focus on delivering care through a range of activities; and expected outcomes, which focuses on the effects of person-centred nursing. The framework is described as a mid-range theory (see Chapter 2).

Nolan et al. (2004) considered the current changes in policy and the emphasis that is being placed on the promotion of person-centred care, which has become a watchword for good practice. Nolan suggests that a relationship-centred approach to care might be more appropriate and argues that a vision of person-centred care that involves respect for personhood is essential. Nolan advocates the senses framework, which was initially developed as a means of providing a rationale for care within institutional settings. The framework creates a sense of security, belonging, continuity, purpose, achievement and significance, and such senses are seen as prerequisites for relationships. The senses framework was developed using interactive focus groups and workshops with practitioners, carers and older people.

It is clear from the discussion above that there has been recent research to advance nursing knowledge in the field of gerontological nursing; however, this has not always been the case, and the next section will look at traditional nursing of older people.

Looking back at the past: traditions of older people's nursing

Person-centred care is advocated as being important to the older person's wellbeing. A humanistic view considers each human being as unique and respects the differences between people (Portner, 2008). The traditions of nursing older people historically lies in the 'Poor Law nurses' of the workhouse infirmaries who worked with chronically sick, bedridden patients and thus took on the stigma of the workhouse, these patients being a low-status group. The 'Poor Law nurses' became known as the 'geriatric nurses'. The speciality of geriatrics, as it was once termed, began in the 1930s, marking the beginning of the development of the curative aspects of care for older people. Despite this, doctors working with older people were often considered inferior in status to those in other specialities since treatment and cure were regarded as the goal of the medical model (Tudor-Hart, 1988). However, after the Second World War there was a growing realisation of the social and medical implications of an ageing population. The Beveridge Report (1942) was the first social planning document to recognise the importance of the problems of older people. Prolonged exposure to institutionalised care was beginning to be recognised as leading to increased physical and mental dependency (Goffman, 1961). Goffman discussed institutionalised care in relation to such characteristics as rigidity of routine; block treatment of staff; depersonalisation of residents; and social distancing between staff and patients.

Traditionally, nursing was seen as an assisting profession to medicine (Baker, 1978; Evers, 1981). Geriatric nursing within the nursing profession itself was often seen as the 'Cinderella' – not as technical as other specialities and not well regarded for career prospects. It was the work of Norton (1975), who investigated the problems of geriatric nursing in hospitals and reported research studies of patients and nurses' work, which highlighted ritualistic practice based on routine rather than need.

The study conducted by Wells in 1980 was aimed at describing current nursing practice in order to develop a potential model for geriatric nursing. Wells concluded at that time that the environment posed many problems, and that nurses lacked the understanding and knowledge necessary to cope with the nursing problems of their patients in order to promote change. Nurses often showed a lack of awareness about current practice together with a lack of planning and communication:

> The nursing work on the geriatric wards was not focused on the patient needs but on ward routines, which might or might not be appropriate for each patient. The work routines were based on minimal, universal needs such as meals, commoding, changing wet pads, getting up and going to bed. Work was not organised in the sense that it was assigned in any manner. Routines were determined by the time of day and the work progressed in bursts of frantic activity by nurses working in pairs or a group of three to complete the routine from one end of the ward to another. Further, not only was work not assigned or even focused on individual patients but there was no nursing record of individual patient preference and no such information was transmitted verbally in nurse communication. Moreover, individual patient preference or even necessary variation in care appeared to be obstructive to the work goal, which was completion of routine. Thus, the problem of nursing work in geriatric wards was not so much shortage of staff as the fact that such work was neither sensibly organised nor provided the likelihood of helpful care for patients. Patients' physical care problems were not a central issue. Nursing staff were not concerned about any specific patient problem; their prime concern was the completion of ward routines. (Wells, 1980: 128)

The disadvantages that nurses and older people had to cope with during this time were not highlighted. This, of course, does not excuse poor nursing care, but could have helped to explain the constraints and circumstances of nurses' work at that time. Baker (1978) researched the relationship between nurses' perceptions of their work and actual work behaviour. Baker's research indicated that patients were not treated as adults, and nursing care was routine and not individualised at all.

'Geriatrics' was seen as a difficult area in nursing due to the patients' multiple health problems. It is recognised that a single diagnosis is frequently impossible in older people as they usually present with multi-pathology involving the ageing process. In addition to the physical aspects of medicine, social situations and home circumstances need to be considered. Historically, the focus of traditional medicine and nursing has been on the treatment of disease. There has, however, been a growing interest in the organisation of nursing in terms of patient-centred care, which has helped to focus attention on the individual needs of hospitalised older people (RCN, 2006). This approach recognises that older people are consumers of care and the focus of nursing is to enable the individual to maximise and adapt according to their potential, within various settings.

A number of studies have reported that many nurses are not interested in working within care of the older people (Melanson and Downe-Wamboldt, 1985; Dellasega and Curriero, 1991; Slevin, 1991; Stevens and Crouch, 1992; Pursey and Luker, 1995; Herdman, 2002; Nolan et al., 2004). These studies have suggested that there exist attitudes of ageism in society, with age-related views and prejudices. When studying nurses working with older people, Pursey and Luker (1995) found that organisation of work and structural locations of older people's care were aspects prompting frustration and stress in nurses, not necessarily the patients themselves. This is the case not only in the United Kingdom; in Sweden, for example, Fagerberg's (1998) doctoral study investigated nursing students' narrated lived experiences of caring, education and the transition into nursing, focusing on areas of older people's nursing.

The majority of the students preferred to work in emergency care rather than older people's care, after graduation. Nurses' attitudes towards working with older people have reflected negative stereotypes of old age in society. There has seemed to be a stigma attached to working with older people. Care of older people is seen as an unpopular choice for students and has not been viewed as an academic area to study or to work in. The nursing literature is replete with reports of nursing negativity and attitudes in relation to older people (Herdman, 2002; Murray, 2002). This creates a paradox inasmuch as older people have the greatest need for nursing services but evidence seems to suggest that fewer nurses are seeking to work with older people as a career option.

This creates something akin to Tudor-Hart's 1988 inverse care law. Older people have the greatest need for nursing and medical services and yet care of older people has been low in the priority of policy makers and in medical and nursing services themselves. Tudor-Hart concluded that care of older people involves even more people than care of the dying and with less help from the NHS and other social agencies. Tudor-Hart gave an example of informal carers who could not go out to work, their families and their lives being disrupted for months – even years – and then they may become socially isolated and exhausted, and are often sick or old themselves.

Nurses working in care of older people have challenged attitudes and current methods of nursing assessment (RCN, 2004), which has resulted in greater autonomy and clarified something of the nature of expert practice. Such a trend has enabled developments whereby person-centred nursing has become more widely accepted.

From the nursing literature (RCN, 2006), the nurse's role in care of older people has been seen to involve:

promoting the physical and emotional health of older people;
helping them to maintain their independence;
providing effective treatments;
facilitating rehabilitation;
responding to more complex care needs;
arranging effective continuing health and palliative care.

Portner (2008) suggests that the primary motivation for all service developments with older people must be the need to improve the quality of care the older person receives. This means questioning the nurse's role and function in working with older people. Nolan (2004) advocates that efforts to develop a knowledge base to guide nursing practice in care of older people should abandon the search for grand theories and focus instead on building a core of practice theory which is of relevance to all those working with older people.

In 2004 the Royal College of Nursing produced its strategy to promote the contribution nurses can make for older people. The report established a vision for care of older people and gave information regarding good nursing practice. The themes of the strategy that underpin nursing practice are:

valuing older people;
maximising potential;
ensuring good-quality physical, mental and emotional care;
enabling information sharing with older people and their carers;
working in partnership with older people.

In acute secondary care in the United Kingdom's Health Service there has been an integration of geriatric medicine with the acute medical services. Whilst there remain some valid arguments for the concept of integrated services for older people, there are still perceived benefits in providing specialist environments. An on-line survey called 'Dignity in Care' (DoH, 2006) spoke directly to the public about their experiences of being treated. Some issues that arose from the survey related to:

lack of clarity about what standards to expect;
difficulty in making a complaint;
people not being listened to or treated as individuals;
not enough assistance, insufficient access to toilets/bathrooms;
being placed in mixed-sex facilities and being made to feel uncomfortable;
lack of privacy when receiving care. (DoH, 2006)

The *National Service Framework for Older People* (DoH, 2001) has been part of a standard-setting framework that targets chronic diseases, and has evolved out of the need to improve the efficiency, effectiveness and services for older people. The National Service Framework (NSF) is a strategy that was set to ensure high-quality, integrated health and social care services for older people. In its ten-year programme, it is intended to link services to support independence and to promote good health, provide specialist services for key conditions, and develop a culture change working towards respect, dignity and fairness. The NSF sets out an agenda to improve standards and to reduce unacceptable variations in health and social services. It focuses on:

rooting out discrimination;
providing person-centred care;
promoting older people's health and independence;
fitting services around people's needs.

The NHS for older people addresses those conditions that are particularly related to older people, for example stroke, falls and mental health problems associated with old age.

Health and social care in the community

More and more people in the United Kingdom are surviving to old age and this has been one of the biggest achievements of the twentieth century. In an ideal world, old age would be accompanied by adequate finances and adequate fitness. However, in practice, the maintenance of good health in older people requires active help by health practitioners in preventing ill health and providing the appropriate level of support. It seems that current health and social policy has a greater impact on older people and their receipt of effective services. In addition, it is generally assumed that the increasing number of older people is resulting in greater demands being placed on healthcare resources.

Nurses are involved in assessment of older people in primary and secondary care. Practice nurses in surgeries as well as district nurses are responsible for the annual health check for people aged 75 years and over and were introduced into Primary Health care in the UK as part of the General Medical Contract. However, although some areas of assessment are identified in the contract, there does not appear to be a standardised assessment tool in use.

Shifting boundaries

Good health is seen as a key issue in quality of life amongst older people. Access to good healthcare is considered along with such issues as dignity, privacy, independence, choice, rights and fulfilment. However, there is still concern about the quality of care provided not only to the older person but also their carers (Nolan et al., 1995; Davies and Nolan, 2006). Outside the National Health Service there have been major changes in community care which have resulted in an attempt to deliver a seamless service between health and social care. What was once seen as district nursing, for example such skills as washing, dressing and mobilising, has now been reclassified as social care. These shifting boundaries between health and social care, together with the speciality of gerontological nursing and the more general care of the older person, make the identification of nursing care of the older person more complex.

These shifting boundaries have masked the increasing number of older people who need acute hospitalised intense nursing care, in terms of their potential to be rehabilitated. Indeed, the number and type of agencies involved in the assessment, planning, delivery and evaluation of services are increasing. Care of the older person is thus influenced by the context in which the care is given. Likewise, nursing is one of many components of healthcare for older people. Apart from the immense changes that are occurring within strategic service developments, there have been developments within the nursing profession itself.

Front-line role models: nurses

Nursing, like other professional groups, is affected by wider sociological and political assumptions relating to old age. As such, much of the United Kingdom in the past has been seen to be ageist, with older people commonly portrayed as an insupportable burden on the welfare state. Nurses are seen as front-line role models of the National Health Service and could help to change these attitudes. It is understandable that many older people have mixed feelings and apprehension about healthcare and admission into hospital, which can create feelings of fear and uncertainty about the future. The Department of Health NHS Improvement Plan (2004) suggested, from listening to older people, that they want health and social services that will put them, and their needs and wishes, at the centre of service delivery whether in secondary or primary care.

In primary care, community nursing services are using the Evercare programme, which has been developed in America to improve the quality of life for older people in primary care. Evercare involves developing new ways of working for healthcare professionals and is now being introduced into many Primary Care Trusts within the UK. The focus is on helping older people to maintain their independence, improve their wellbeing and avoid the need to go into hospital. Case management is seen as a way to improve the quality of care and help the older person to make choices in their management. Self-care is seen as part of daily living: it is care taken by the individual towards their own health and wellbeing in order to stay fit and to maintain good physical and mental health, meet social and psychological needs, prevent illness or to care for long-term conditions. Evercare is a different approach to care in the community but it also requires a different style of nurse practitioner to encourage patients to be more independent.

Conclusion

In order to become more focused on the theory on which nurses base their practice, Morse (1995) suggests a qualitative framework that uses actual clinical data to develop concepts of nursing, and suggests an inductive approach to theory building and concept development. Such an inductive approach would not seek to test hypotheses but rather to describe and explain the world of nursing. This form of theory development, acknowledging the social world in which nursing takes place, could therefore be more immediately relevant to nursing than abstract grand theories (Smith, 1992; Savage, 1995). Charmaz (2006) suggests a move towards grounded theory in nursing to develop theories relevant to older people's practice. Charmaz advocates grounded theory as the combination of involvement and interpretation that leads the researcher to take the next steps in developing practice. Charmaz talks of the end point of the researcher's journey: it emerges from where you start, where you go, and with whom you interact, what you see and hear, and how you learn and think.

This was the approach taken by the author to research care of older people presented in this book. The next chapter looks at the care of older people and the settings in which nursing care takes place; in addition, the author discusses the care of older people in hospitalised settings.

Suggested reading

Ghaye, T. and Lillyman, S., eds. (2000) *Caring Moments – The Discourse of Reflective Practice* (Wiltshire: The Cromwell Press). This is a book within a series on reflective practice. The book looks at the strength of storytelling in healthcare. The stories look at the details of clinical and caring practice, and illuminate complex issues such as the self, experience, career, identity, expectation, contradiction, spirituality, agency and social culture.

Hill, M. (2003) *Understanding Social Policy*, 7th edition (Oxford: Blackwell Publishing). This book looks at the new and strengthened policy linkages. It examines the way that social policy has been transformed by changes in politics and society.

Jamieson, A. and Victor, C., eds. (2002) *Researching Ageing and Later Life* (London: Open University Press). This edited volume addresses the methodological challenges entailed in studying the process of ageing and life course changes, and the experience of being old. The book focuses on the theory and practice of doing research using a wide range of case studies.

Symonds, A. and Kelly, A. (1998) *The Social Construction of Community Care* (Basingstoke: Macmillan Press). This book represents a new development in the discussion of community care policies and their implementation as it attempts an integrated overview. The book applies a sociological perspective of community and social care.

Warnes, A., Warren, L. and Nolan, M. (2000) *Care Services for Later Life* (London: Jessica Kingsley Publishers). This book examines the implications of current economic social and political trends in Britain for older people. The authors take a critical look at the current situation and assess the implications for future practice.

Part II

Research and practice

Chapter 4

The context and culture of the care setting

This chapter:

▶ describes care of older people in primary and secondary care;
▶ discusses the wards in which the study in this book took place.

Part II of this book describes the detail of nursing care that the author encountered. It shows aspects of nursing coined by the term 'just basic nursing care' and often taken-for-granted aspects within nursing. The practice theory within 'basic nursing care' has not been regarded as 'formal knowledge' and the author could not always find any textbook knowledge to describe this, because of the unique and individual nature of each experience. The author has put together the practice theories into a framework for the practice of care of older people, which could serve as a good yardstick to measure or to guide nursing care of older people. The author draws on the words of the nurses, which show the complexity of nursing and the ways in which nurses manage this. We begin by looking at the general future practice and long-term care of older people, outlining the philosophy of this nursing care; this will be followed, in Chapter 5, by a discussion of the framework used.

A changing approach to policies for care of older people

Over the next 20 years demographic changes will significantly alter the balance of the population and therefore the balance of the NHS and healthcare; policy will need to reflect the needs of an ageing society. This is to say that there will be a need to improve the quality, quantity and responsiveness of the NHS and social care for older people. Over the last five years a large number of policies have been developed with the overarching aim of improving older people's lives. Some of these promote independence and wellbeing, such as the *National Service Framework for Older People* (DoH, 2001), with standards tackling age discrimination and others promoting health and active life. It seems that services for older people have traditionally focused on the most at risk older person, and have tended to be reactive in times of crisis, rarely going beyond the crisis problems towards life-long health in a holistic way for each individual. Future policies and standards will go beyond a reactive model to a proactive approach which will focus on *all* older people's needs, continually assisting independence and wellbeing. It is hoped that future care of older people will be guided by the following principles produced in the 2004 Audit Commission Report:

▶ providing increased choice and control;
▶ promoting healthy lifestyles;
▶ adopting a 'whole person' approach;
▶ building a 'whole system' response.

This new way of working in government strategy should result in:

▶ fewer hospital admissions;
▶ shorter average lengths of stay;
▶ reduction in visits to accident and emergency departments;
▶ less use of GP services.

This should reduce pressure on acute hospitals.

Acute secondary hospital care

The management and care of older patients in the acute setting has become a high priority for the NHS. There is an urgent need to reduce the number of emergency beds used by older people, who are admitted to hospital with chronic and long-term conditions. Quite apart from the quality of life issues for the older person and their carers, there is also the impact on the acute hospital settings in terms of service demands (Kings Fund, 2004). The main challenge is that older individuals consume the largest proportion of health and social care resources, and these need to be reduced in the future.

There is an overall government strategy looking at health issues in the broader sense as they relate to older people, and considering how they affect the rest of the community. The report *Better Health in Old Age*, produced by the Department of Health in 2004, suggests that pressure of acute care has been growing partly because of a rise in emergency medical admissions, with the result that older people are being admitted to acute areas. Given these increases, acute hospitals are reducing the length of stay to increase their throughput. Clearly, shorter lengths of stay make it more difficult to plan discharges. Some older patients are therefore readmitted with many of the same problems they had on previous hospitalisation. Whilst most patients are eager to return home after hospital care, some may still require rehabilitation.

Pause for thought

Whether you are a nurse working in surgery, medicine or orthopaedic nursing, what is the ratio of older patients that you care for? How much of your time is spent dealing with discharge issues?

In addition, policy shifts have resulted in an increasing emphasis on convalescence, rehabilitation and intermediate care. The government's White Paper *The New NHS* (DoH, 1997) emphasised a commitment to rehabilitation services as a way of emphasising the importance of rehabilitation in the health service. The nursing-home care sector, in particular, is shifting its emphasis away from residential focus to that of rehabilitation. Such a divide has enabled the reduction of healthcare commitment to the support of older people throughout their lives and in particular the erosion of continuing care, residential and primary services.

With an ageing population the burden on healthcare is continually increasing and there are major social care implications as well. Currently, chronic diseases are amongst the costliest to treat, and account for around a third of emergency admissions to NHS beds in the over-65 age group. The DoH (2007) suggests in its report *A Recipe for Care – Not a Single Ingredient* that older people are three times more likely than younger people to be admitted to hospital following attendance at an Emergency Department. Older people might have more than one long-term condition and are often taking a mixture of medications. This in itself can lead to problems such as falls and confusion. To cope with these issues key elements are advised:

1. Early intervention and assessment of old age conditions.
2. Long-term conditions managed in the community and integrated with social care and specialist services.
3. Early supported discharge whenever possible, delivering care close to home.
4. General acute hospital care whenever needed combined with quick access to out-of-hour services. Partnership built around the needs and wishes of older people and their families. (DoH, 2007: 1)

In the UK, chronic illness is the single largest cause of poor health, and makes the greatest use of healthcare resources. Acute episodes of conditions such as heart failure, diabetes and respiratory problems account for admission into acute hospital beds. This is a growing problem and the NHS and social communities are finding it difficult to meet demand.

Proactive approaches are being devised and are intended to bring benefits to older people, as well as to the wider NHS and social care system. In the future, people with long-term conditions will have their needs met by an extended primary care team who will be working with the voluntary sector and carers. Admission to hospital will happen as part of agreed care pathways. There are going to be immense changes in the future care of older people, and there will be greater opportunity than at the present for community nurses to meet the challenges in primary care settings. There are opportunities through expert patient groups and greater patient participation to enable lay people to become expert leaders of expert groups. It is anticipated that community nurses are going to be the leaders of that type of care but there has to be improved accessibility for patients to services.

Working across secondary and primary care services

The policy vision will demand a change of thinking both from the public and the collaborative approach in primary care in order to be effective and to prevent diseases. Community nurses don't work in isolation; they work across boundaries through health and social care, linking with groups such as housing, environment issues, public health, and health visitors, and working closely with other members of the medical profession towards preventative medicine.

In the UK, 60 per cent of hospital beds are filled with people with long-term conditions. It is estimated that 17.5 million adults in the UK are living with chronic conditions, with people over the age of 65 being most affected. However, the DoH is estimating that this figure will double by the year 2030, so there are immense challenges and opportunities for future care of older people.

The only answer, then, is to move away from reactive care based in acute systems towards routine care in primary care – working in partnership across the whole of health and social care so that healthcare is shifted towards primary care. Figure 4.1 illustrates the range of staff across the various sectors – health, social care and the voluntary sector – that are engaging with the long-term management of older people.

Nursing older people is about developing a self-care model which in turn involves the teaching and education of older people and their carers. This should not mean the giving of information in a didactic way; it should be by demonstrating and showing older people how to self-manage and giving them practical help. Resource centres with teams of people – i.e. advanced nurse practitioners, district nurses and practice nurses – will be able to get involved with families and carers in an innovative way.

Nurses need to consider the social and cultural aspects of care and the relationship between health and social care so that they will have a map of the care pathway for the older person.

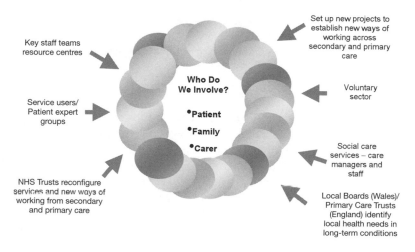

Figure 4.1   Staff engaging with the long-term management of older people

Older people's nursing in primary care

Care of older people is definitely in the limelight of government policies (DoH, 2006). Evidence suggests there are ongoing issues facing many older people living in the community in the United Kingdom, issues such as age discrimination, stereotyping, poor engagement with younger people, social exclusion, isolation, poverty. Gaps of understanding exist between the various generations, older people having endured war, the hardship of food rationing and having to make ends meet in their earlier lives. Now, many of those people are over 80 and having to endure social and financial difficulties, some hardly managing to pay their winter heating bills.

However, older people are an asset to the community; in many cultures and communities, they play a significant part in family life. They also have a wealth of knowledge and experience that can be of benefit to the community and primary care. Despite this, however, in our society older people are often regarded as a burden and of less value than younger people.

It is clear that many older people are struggling to cope with chronic and long-term conditions on a day-to-day basis in the community. Despite our progress in technology in healthcare, it seems that the basic factors needed to achieve good health in older people remain the same. Housing, health and social care services are essential to allowing the older person to remain independent.

Pause for thought

What are the major issues for community nursing regarding caring for older people in your area?

Delivering Care, Enabling Health (Scottish Executive, 2006) has signalled a fundamental shift from a service that is focused on providing hospital care to one where care is planned closer to home, making community nursing more proactive within primary care. Clearly community nurses are at the heart of health services, working in partnership with individuals, carers, families, communities and professional services. Community nurses are the very essence of the delivery of 'tailor made', high-quality services for those individuals who need them.

Case management's broad aim is to develop cost-effective and efficient ways of co-ordinating services. It is a way forward for delivering holistic healthcare matched to the older person with complex health and social care needs. Within a case management approach there is an increased emphasis on nurse-led case management, where the district nurse will focus on clinical needs with the aim of minimising symptoms of the medical condition, thus preventing admission to hospital. Of course, dealing with the medical problem alone will not achieve this; the combination of heath, social and maybe other services will need to be activated as well. Figure 4.2 shows the aims of remodelling care of older people in primary care.

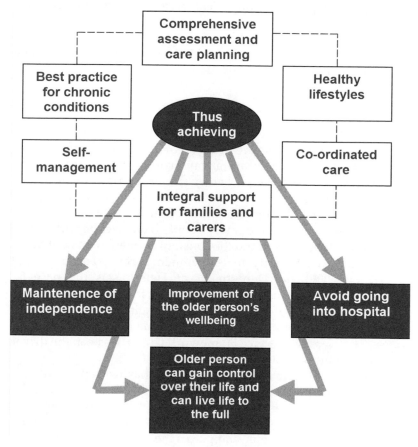

Figure 4.2   Aims of remodelling care of older people in primary care

Clearly, people in the twenty-first century expect services to be fast, high quality, responsive and fitted around their lives (DoH, 2006). As a public service, the nursing of older people should be about the person, as nursing care is personal to them. In essence, care and nursing support in the community should enable older people to make the most of their lives.

The government White Paper (DoH, 2006) has a strategy for all the care and support services that people use in their communities and has three themes for future care:

▶ putting people more in control of their own health and care;
▶ enabling and supporting health independence and wellbeing;
▶ providing rapid and convenient access to high-quality, cost-effective care.

Community nurses, in caring for older people, will be refocusing their care in a new direction.

Informal carers of older people

It seems that almost every day there are media reports about care of older people. Alarm bells are being sounded about standards and quality of care and there are always comments regarding how older people are cared for, whether they are in a nursing home, hospital or living at home (Smith, 2006; Froggatt et al., 2009). Stories good or bad hit the headlines. What is least reported is the day-to-day way in which ordinary people have to cope with caring for a failing older relative and the constant burden to them of informal care in the community. In its document *A New Ambition for Old Age* (DoH, 2006), the Department of Health sets the pace by addressing key challenges for the future. It identifies the need for older people to be treated with respect for their dignity and human rights in all care settings, whether at home, in hospital or care homes. The National Service Framework (2001) has been the driver of many advances in terms of these issues.

Health promotion and elective healthcare has, as well as reducing delayed discharge from hospital, increased the proportion of older people with high levels of need remaining in their own homes for longer. The NSF has gone a long way to changing the culture towards care of older people and places the needs of older people at the centre of care.

Pause for thought

It is worth taking note of the feelings and attitudes of people in general as to how they would like to be cared for when they are older – or, more to the point, what you would want when you are older.

Have you ever thought about getting old? How it might feel? What you might be like? How you would maintain your dignity and pride?

The King's Fund study (2005) explored the attitudes of people in their fifties now, from a range of backgrounds, to find out how they would like to be cared for and where they would want to live when they are older. It is very clear from that study that most people wanted to 'live their own lives' and did not want to be cared for by their children. The majority of people interviewed wanted to remain independent and continue with their type of 'modern' lifestyle when they are older. It seems there was less worry about personal care or nursing care. However, they requested the need for more help with domestic work and heavy lifting.

Generally, those interviewed want to 'have a life' in old age; they did not want to stop enjoying themselves just because they were old, nor did they want to be dependent on anyone. They wanted less emphasis on nursing care and more on being cared for in the form of plenty of help with domestic work.

Pause for thought

▶ What sort of lifestyle do you want when you are older?
▶ Where do you want to live?
▶ Who will care for you?

According to the Carers National Association, there are 6.8 million carers in the United Kingdom, one in every seven adults being a carer in the community. In the UK, a great deal of care of older people is informally provided by their spouses and by their children, friends and voluntary organisations at little financial cost to the government. Care assistance includes social, emotional, physical and often technical care. With the progressive increase in dependency from the older person, help with activities of daily living (ADL) such as bathing, dressing, mobility, toileting or eating also becomes necessary. Successful living in the community also entails ADL in the form of shopping, cooking, housework, banking, transport, management of medications. All of these activities are time intensive and can add significantly to the stress generated by care giving regardless of the age of the informal care giver.

Care of older people in hospital

In the study reported on in this book the nurses worked in hospital wards. The three wards studied were fairly typical in design of most National Health Service acute older people's wards and all were managed under the same NHS trust. Two wards were within a small community hospital approximately two miles away from the main District General Hospital, whilst the third was within the acute hospital. Patient admission to the older people's wards included direct admission from home via the general practitioner, transfers for patients requiring rehabilitation following surgery, transfers from private and residential nursing settings and direct admissions from the Emergency Departments. The wards thus contained a mix of acutely ill older patients, together with the more intermediate-care patients requiring a rehabilitation process. All three wards were 28-bed wards with mixed male and female patients. Each of the wards had a mixture of individual side rooms and there were also six-bed bays down one side of the ward used mainly for patients undergoing rehabilitation and intermediate care.

Each ward had a sister in charge, with another acting as the second sister in charge. There were student nurses in undergraduate studies allocated to the wards. The two wards situated in the smaller community hospital were light and airy with ample space for the family to sit and for relatives to take a break. Both the wards had very large dayrooms which also served as dining areas, with large picture windows and doors leading out onto a patio area. There was a particularly homely atmosphere in these rooms, which contained a television, music, and lots of photos, plants and activities. In addition, there was usually some occupational therapy or other activity going on.

Issues relating to the maintenance of standards was directly linked to the nurses' management role and being in charge of the ward. Nurses were key figures in the overall management of the ward and discussed continuity of care as a major issue. They were a constant source of information for all staff and visitors since they were the only members of the multidisciplinary team constantly within the ward. They remained with the patients for the duration of their span of duty, a fact which gave them every opportunity to be responsible and in charge of the patient care.

Two of the wards observed agreed to a system of nurse-managed beds. These beds were managed by nurse practitioners who were the named nurses. A number of nurses in the literature have argued that a need exists for the provision of nurse-managed beds in particular specialties that focus on the delivery of therapeutic nursing. Nursing beds are essentially those established where nursing is the chief therapy and the nurse is the chief therapist. They are based on the fundamental belief that nursing in itself can be therapeutic.

Patients nursed in these beds required high nursing interventions with low medical intervention. The protocol was for the local General Practitioner service to be utilised if required for medical advice. Protocols of referral were also in place for the nurses to refer the patient to the medical staff if required to do so.

The nurses supported individual nursing because they felt that it enabled the nurses to communicate better with the patients and their families. The multidisciplinary team were then able to identify with the patient's own nurse. The nurses stressed that primary nursing gave them greater autonomy and responsibility.

There were great opportunities to develop nursing practice in caring for older people by working across boundaries with health and social care staff and, indeed, with families and relatives. Management of long-term conditions is identified as a key area in the health and social policy agenda; it has created major opportunities for nurses to take the lead and to work innovatively with families and at a community public health level.

Care of the hospitalised older person in its broader context referred to economic, professional and philosophical issues that have significant impact on the relationship between the nurse and the patient, along with the more focused individual care. Many hospital admissions in this clinical area were necessitated by inadequate social support rather than a medical condition. For many, admission into hospital represented deteriorating health, and loss of independence, social contact and personal identity. Older people in the acute hospital setting seemed especially prone to a unique set of problems. The early identification of problems such as confusion, urinary incontinence and falling can greatly affect the patient's rehabilitation in the context of this setting.

Nursing care for the older person involves a particular type of nurse–patient relationship that enables growth and recovery of potential. The therapeutic approach undertaken emphasises the need to develop the future potential of the older person. The nurses observed in the study displayed their ability to equip the older person with new skills and enable them to be self-caring. Although many professional disciplines contribute to the healthcare of older people, the day-to-day care rested mainly with the nursing staff. Nursing the older person was centrally about equipping them with skills to care for themselves.

Nursing the older person is fraught with social dilemmas not least because the nurses are dealing with people who are particularly vulnerable. Older patients are often depressed, for example following bereavement, as well as being frail and unable to look after themselves and possibly having little motivation. Older people's nursing is difficult; there are many issues of concern and the nurse needs to understand the social background of the patient in order to conceptualise how the patient's ill health and disease process will affect their lifestyle. The majority of nurses demonstrated a very well-informed account of their patients as people, often discussing the smallest detail about the home condition and social setting.

Nurses seemed to be able to respond rapidly in changing situations. This may have been in relation to an aspect of physical care; sometimes it was by responding to verbal interactions with patients. The nurses were allocated as named nurses to their patients; there was very often a sense of a special relationship between the nurse and patient. The nurses seemed really interested in their patients and showed a genuine desire for the patients to want to get better.

Many of the nurses were dealing with unique situations where they responded by drawing on their experiences and selecting an approach to a particular individual situation based on a wide range of previous experiences in that area of practice. Elliott (1991), discussing practical wisdom, referred to the practitioners' capacity to take the right course of action when faced with particular complex situations. Elliott referred to practical wisdom or knowledge as knowing how to act in relation to circumstances of a particular situation or context.

It was interesting to explore how nurses gained understanding and became involved with the families of older patients. There was a major effort by the nurses to develop a working relationship which was mainly achieved through interacting with the relatives. This was usually done at the bedside through talking, explaining and responding in practice. Of course, family-focused care has long been espoused by professional nurses as desirable (Reed, 2006).

Effective nursing care was demonstrated by enhancing the nurse–patient relationship through informal interactions and companionship. The aim was to increase family resources through multidisciplinary assessments of activities of daily living and to increase families' informal care-giving skills by open visiting and participation in care. The nurses demonstrated in their interactions and by responding rapidly to the patients that their role was facilitation of the transition back home.

Many of the nurses talked about the needs of the family as being a crucial issue in older people's nursing. Nolan et al. (2004) suggest that professionals adopt a 'carers as experts' model in which the primary aim of interventions is to assist users to acquire the skills and competencies they need. Carers often have to cope with problems themselves due to a delay in receiving professional help. There is a recognition of new carers as novices who are expected to provide complex physical care and to make far-reaching decisions without adequate preparation.

Conclusion

The nurses had a working philosophy of care that they felt was underpinning their practice:

> To us the most important aspect of nursing is caring, with the aim to accept people and to know them as individuals. By doing this we can provide comfort, support and enhance a client's independence and dignity. We actively encourage the involvement of families and close friends in client care. In order to work together effectively for the benefit of our clients, the multidisciplinary team depends on effective communication. Each individual has the right to be assessed by a skilled professional and to agree to the planning of the programme of care. We also need to provide relevant information to promote a healthy lifestyle and give advice on local voluntary organisations and support groups. (Philosophy of nursing care as stated by the ward nursing team)

Older people's nursing was about a more individual perspective towards the patients, their families and the nurse's personal use of self to develop a nurse–patient relationship. It is not only the physical aspects of practice which

Conclusion cont'd

nurses had to consider but also the social, political and economic aspects. The nurses encountered complex problems which could have complicated the discharge process, such as rehousing, admission to a nursing home or residential setting. In addition, the skills required by the trained nurses in older people's nursing care emphasise the importance of assessment and forward planning. The nurses were guided by the philosophy stated above and were able to engage with the family so as to work with them and help them achieve their personal goals.

The assessment process in place demonstrated the important need for nursing knowledge about the older patient, in terms of who they are, where they live and with whom, their current heath status and lifestyle, and their hopes and needs for the future.

Suggested reading

Bowling, A. (2005) *Ageing with Quality of Life in Old Age* (Buckingham: Open University Press).

Froggatt, K., Davis, S. and Meyer, J. (2009) *Understanding Care Homes – A Research and Development Perspective* (London: Jessica Kingsley).

Lawler, J. (1991) *Behind the Screens: Nursing, Somology and the Problems of the Body* (London: Churchill Livingstone). This is a book about nursing that every nurse can identify with. It sheds light on fundamental aspects of basic nursing. The invisibility of nursing is linked with the lack of academic discourse on body care.

Nay, R. and Garratt, S. (2004) *Nursing Older People: Issues and Innovations*, 2nd edition (Australia: Elsevier). Reflects recent changes and developments at a national and international level. The book draws on research undertaken by the authors and gives ideas on ongoing research and development necessary for quality aged care.

Nolan, M., Davies, S. and Grant, G. (2001) *Working with Older People: Key Issues in Policy and Practice* (Buckingham: Open University Press). This book discusses the needs of older people and their carers, an essential element of both policy and practice. The notion of person-centred care is a major feature in this text.

Peckham, S. and Exworthy, M. (2003) *Primary Care in the UK: Policy, Organisation and Management* (Basingstoke: Palgrave Macmillan). This book presents a two-way dialogue between research and policy in primary care. It seeks to offer students, researchers, practitioners and policy makers insights from across the interface.

Chapter 5

A framework for the delivery of care

This chapter:

identifies the framework of practice theory for older people;
looks closely at the features identified within the framework of care.

The framework of care delivery

This chapter aims to look more closely at the framework for the delivery of care for an older person, which has emerged from the author's own research. Her observations of everyday nursing care demonstrated that there were factors of practice theory that seemed to be embedded within the care given to older people. Figure 5.1 shows the main categories and themes that were seen in the first stage of the research analysis. Figure 5.2 identifies the factors in stage two.

The role of the older people's nurse

Nurses identified older people's nursing as 'meeting comfort needs of the patient'. This seems to reflect the notion of 'nursing as nurturing' and 'nursing as nourishing'. Nurturing as nursing is an aspect of nursing care which enabled the older person to feel better about their situation, more comfortable and better able to cope. Building a close nurse–patient relationship enabled this process to happen (see Figure 5.2).

The factors identified were closely related to the notion of nurturing as the purpose of nursing care. Their existence, however, was deeply embedded in the practice of the nurses, sometimes only visible through observation of that practice.

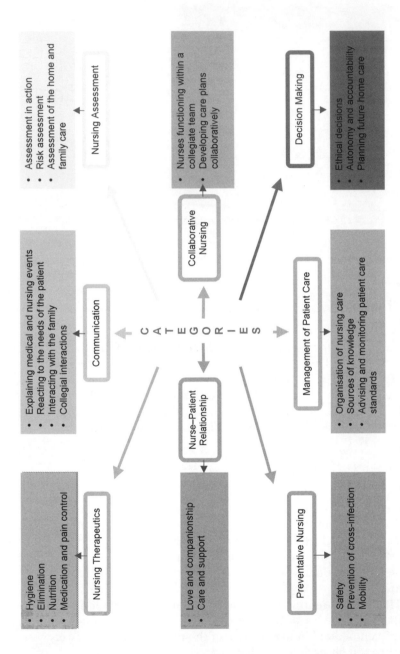

Figure 5.1   Themes and categories of caring for an older person as seen in practice

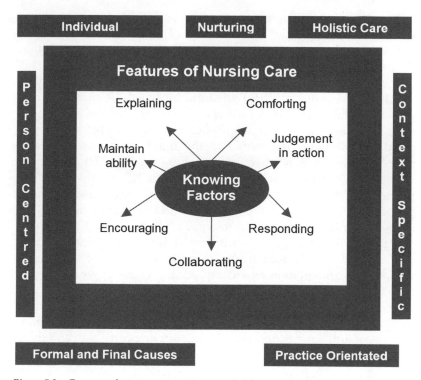

Figure 5.2   Common features present in care of older people

At times, the nurturing aspects of nursing care became overshad-owed by the technical interventions and the nurses themselves downplayed the nurturing aspects of their role, often referring to this simply as 'good nursing care'.

There was a lack of academic literature about these issues to explain what it takes to make an older patient comfortable, or how to give them the will to want to live and look after themselves in terms of maintaining their ability to be self-caring. Despite this, the nurses knew what to do, and displayed this in their 'theories in action'.

In this framework of practice the practice theories appeared as elements of unarticulated practice theory, as it was not always possi-ble to locate that practice in the nursing literature on older people. Sometimes they were mentioned within other concepts in a broad and general way, whereas in practice these factors are patient focused and extremely specific.

The knowledge identified appeared as hidden knowledge, distinct from formal academic knowledge. The factors identified were knowledge that was gained through a process of personalisation. Personal knowledge in the factors seemed to inform the nurses' judgement and was embedded within their performance. Elliott (1991) talked about practical wisdom, by which he meant nurses' capacity to take the right course of action when meeting with particular, complex and problematic issues in practice. Practitioner personal knowledge is not stored in the mind as sets of theoretical propositions but as a reflective repertoire of cases. Thus practical wisdom is knowing how to act in relation to the circumstances of a particular situation or context. This could involve the use of general propositional theories in the more technical aspects of nursing, but by being contextualised it becomes particularised.

Personal knowledge was integrated into the critical thinking process and used automatically in each nursing care experience, with the documentation as a completing process. If we can accept that the nurses' actions were not random or controlled by others, they did also seem to have a theoretical basis for what they did, inasmuch as their decision making was by means of a critical thinking process of judgements in action during nursing care there and then.

The nurse–patient relationship

Explaining care to the older person

An extremely close relationship existed between the older patients and the nurses, and the latter were able to demonstrate the amount of detail that they had gathered about their patients. Their unique position in being the people with a full understanding of particular patients means that that personal knowledge can be optimised.

'Explaining' was a factor that occurred when the nurses were giving information about the older person's care and future home care. It related to the information which was given to the patient concerning their present lifestyle and wellbeing and what may happen in the future. 'Explaining' was defined as 'The nurses constantly transforming information in a meaningful way.' 'Transforming' was about interpreting to the patient significant information related to their medical and nursing care.

The nurses demonstrated an ability to build a therapeutic relationship with the patient by explaining. There was a noticeable difference between the nurses' activity of 'explaining' and merely 'telling'. 'Telling' would simply have involved a process of giving information in a somewhat prescriptive manner, and this was not observed. The nurses worked closely with the patients and always took time when explaining. Figure 5.3 shows all the features in a framework of nursing care of older people as seen in this study.

The value of providing close companionship with the patient has been noted by a number of authors (Benner and Wrubel, 1989; Ersser and Tutton, 1991). Campbell (1984) discussed the companionship offered by nurses to patients as closeness displayed by a bodily presence that involves 'being with' and not just 'doing to'. Nurses regarded the family and the individual personal profile as being significant and through this emerged a unique nurse–patient relationship. Often the nurses would sit at the beside and talk slowly and directly with the patient. They would frequently hold the patient's hand whilst explaining, which demonstrated this close relationship.

The ability to explain indicated to the researcher that the nurses had a constant source of information – which could possibly have been 'know how' knowledge – to call upon as they imparted important information to the patients and their relatives. The nurses were constantly building on a relationship developed by being with the patients and relatives and establishing a trusting relationship. The process of explaining to patients and the nurses' ability to build a working nurse–patient relationship demonstrated a level of knowledge that was a personal knowing and a form of intuitive and experiential knowledge. Benner and Wrubel (1989) identified this as 'embodied knowledge' and it enabled nurses to act in rapid ways.

The ability of the nurse to explain and hence make treatment more meaningful appeared to help the patients – or the nurses believed it helped – when they discussed their care. The benefits of the nurses' embodied knowledge of explaining and activities were self-evident and need no outcome measures. A nursing value system holds that there is a moral duty to 'explain' to patients rather than 'tell' them about their progress.

The nurse talks to the patient and explains that she is going to clean her mouth. The patient is aphasic but seems to be listening to the nurse by looking and smiling at her. There is a very close nurse–patient rapport.

The nurses answered their patients' questions and provided information on a continual basis. Information on all aspects of care

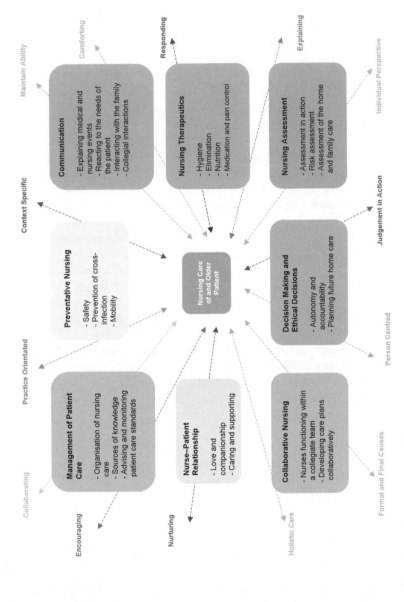

Figure 5.3   Factors in caring for an older person

was often given when personal care was being delivered, such as during bathing, toileting and comforting the patients. Indeed Lawler (1991) referred to this form of knowledge of the body and physical caring and termed it 'somology'. This behaviour by nurses was in complete contrast to the behaviour of other clinicians such as the medical staff, who formalise their information through 'telling the patients' about their treatment during doctors' rounds or during clinics. This was often seen by the patients as authoritative and many did not respond by asking questions.

Most of the nurses spoke to their patients following the doctors' rounds, informing them about the decisions made and allowing time to explain every detail including technical equipment such as intravenous infusions, which often caused the patients anxiety. Can you imagine how frightening the bleeping noise from a naso-gastric feeding pump must be for the older, sensory-impaired patient? However, the author observed occasions where the nurse explained the feeding system and the importance of the feeding regime more than once and was constantly available should the patients need to ask questions. Here is an example of this:

> The nurse sits on the bed and talks to the patient and says his wife will be in later on that evening. She comforts and explains that she is going to change his feed now. The patient tries to pull out the naso-gastric tube ... 'Try not to pull the tube out as it's helping you and feeding you, that's good well done ... The feed is continuously fed down the naso-gastric tube, there nothing to worry about the tube is fine, and the noise is normal, everything is fine. I will make you comfortable now.'

Some nurses explained the reasons for their actions and almost every episode of nursing care began with an explanation to the patient or family member. They would often give an explanation about the purpose of their episode of care and then wait until the patient responded verbally or otherwise before proceeding with the nursing care. Explaining was seen as an ongoing process to enable the patient to be informed about aspects of their care.

> The son was upset and the ward sister took him in her office 'to comfort him' and she explained about the care and rehabilitation his father would be receiving.

This nurse's use of self involved developing a nurse–patient *and* nurse–family relationship by explaining about the care the father would be receiving. The nurse used every opportunity to explain the aspects of care and rehabilitation to the patient, relatives and carers.

Encouragement of the older person

Encouragement was given when the nurses gave direct nursing care and it was mostly conducted in a private way during episodes of nursing care. This often focused on nursing activities such as walking and rehabilitating a patient, mobilising, or attending to the pressure areas or toileting. As was observed from an episode of care:

The patient seems to respond to the encouragement but it has taken a long time to mobilise him. I do not know if he is going to be safe enough to live on his own in the future.

Here the nurse is in the private domain of nursing care, and working with the patient to regain his confidence to walk and be self-caring in the future. Often the nurse would bargain with the patient by giving gentle encouragement because patients were often reluctant to walk and generally did not want to become mobile:

I will walk you to the toilet, and then if you are too tired I will bring you back to your bed in a wheelchair.

It was occasions such as these where patients received the skills of nursing care, including motivating and empowering them to maintain or improve their optimum independence.

The nurse explains that the patient is now able to walk with the use of a walking stick but the patient says that she still feels unsteady, the nurse says she encourages her by walking at her side holding her arm and constantly talks and says she is encouraging her to be as mobile as possible.

The nurses often used the term 'encouragement' as a therapeutic aspect of care required. For example, they spoke of 'fluids being encouraged', 'encouraging walking' and 'encouraging feeding'. This is a term that the nurses knew and understood as significant in nursing. Encouragement was a language in nursing that had a meaning within nursing practice. The nurses also discussed the regime of total patient care as encouragement. This was a phrase that was embedded in practice. Interestingly, it is a term that has been discussed in the theoretical literature as one linked to traditional aspects of nursing and is seen as a blanket statement referring to the more routine cares. Gibb and O'Brian (1991) conducted an ethnographic study into conversation styles used by registered nurses with elderly residents during activities of morning care. Speech was analysed and was seen to vary in relation to various physical procedures. This was seen to have an important psychological function which reflected a particular way of relating. There was optimal use of physical activities of nursing care to achieve greatest benefits in relation to the psychological wellbeing of clients achieved through verbal communication. This was similar to the author's findings and supports the practice theory of encouragement isolated in the study in this book.

The patient needs total nursing care and encouragement. She had a brother living in the area and a daughter. The family was marvellous totally supporting of each other.

Despite this, the author searched the literature for detailed accounts of the issue of encouragement in older people's nursing, such as a concept clarification of encouragement, but could not locate this as a significant aspect in the literature. Encouragement was a factor that appeared to be unarticulated in the theoretical literature. Yet these nurses knew how to encourage patients and to motivate them to wellbeing, as well as being rational and thoughtful about their practice. They discussed what encouraging and nursing meant to them. Such ideas could be referred to as action theories, given the fact that these experiences in practice are unique. As such, they remain an untapped source and, as Benner (1984) found in her research, there are many aspects of nursing practice that remain undocumented in the literature.

Encouragement was significant and was referred to as a constant element of patient care. Encouragement was about making the patient feel better and helping them to regain their confidence and motivation to recover. The nurses made it quite clear that the notion of encouragement was very important in their daily practice. It could possibly have been a way of working through difficult situations; despite all the problems facing the patient, there was encouragement and hope that the situation would improve. Schon (1991) argued that there is a growing awareness in professional groups that practice situations are characterised by uncertainty, uniqueness and instability. However, practitioners do act competently in such difficult situations and often relate to their own specialised personal knowledge alone. Practitioners have to deal with the 'wholeness' of the problem. The problems are encountered in the 'swampy lowlands of practice' and as such are not clearly defined. This was the case for these nurses. The literature did not seem to relate to the issues that the nurses were coping with. Indeed, the author wondered if the application of the available techniques for problem solving is ever able to match what practice is about. However, the nurses managed with 'what they knew' and constantly applied this knowing in their daily practice.

Maintaining ability

The maintenance work of older people's nurses was at an individual and personal level and was associated with the preventative aspects of nursing. It was demonstrated in action and only visible to those who chose to observe it or to those patients who were consumers. Rehabilitation looked ordinary and in an era of clinical effectiveness, where all practitioners are being challenged to demonstrate the outcomes of their practice, this can in some ways be a contradiction in terms. An example showing this occurred when a patient was admitted needing mobilisation:

> You see it is not just about helping the patient onto the commode and preventing her falling or injuring herself. I am maintaining her mobility and rehabilitating her, to see if she is improving and able to manage to care for herself and prevent problems of falling.

> I put the commode opposite the patient, that way I could get her to a standing position and then turn her around slowly to maintain her mobility. The patient was able to practise using her right side and prevent her from ignoring her affected side and falling.

The nurse encouraged the patient by walking with her, sitting out of bed and indeed preventing the hazards of bed rest such as pressure sores, infections, constipation, general debility and deterioration. The point here was that the nurse used her knowledge of mobilisation and rehabilitation as well as the constant therapeutic use of self in the nurse–patient relationship to enable the patient to achieve this optimum potential. The outcomes of the nurse's interventions were the ability of the patient to be self-caring and able to look after herself at home and maintain her ability to do this. This was an outcome of nursing care for the older person that has far-reaching consequences for the patient in terms of their quality of life in the future.

Despite the relative importance of this work, it seemed that the nurses had been conditioned into describing this type of nursing care as 'basic'. When questioned, they would make superficial their reasons for their actions. McCormack summed this up by saying that 'Nurses working with older people have always experienced difficulties in articulating the knowledge, skills and expertise underpinning their practice and their impact on nursing care' (2001: 290). Therefore, the virtue of maintenance as preventive nursing goes unrecognised publicly. A nurse washing a patient is seen as a hygiene activity. However, the nurses often discussed the need to encourage patients to do as much for themselves as possible. They discussed assessing movements of the patient and the condition of the skin. All of these issues are important aspects of nursing care which could restore the older patient to being self-caring and prevent problems of immobility.

The theory in action as maintenance was possibly tacit knowledge, as the nurses often made quite superficial explanations regarding their practice. However, when talking during the interviews they described maintaining the patient as self-caring and the establishment of patients' mobility and independence as a principle, which embodies many ethical beliefs about a person's human need to be self-caring. There were problems in defining, describing and making explicit such knowledge known by the nurses since it was seen as an aspect of prevention.

Advising as a constant professional support

Advising was seen as a particular type of way that the nurses used their personal knowledge and showed an ability to use their personal self to impart this information in a nurse–patient relationship.

The nurses advised on decisions relating to home care, which was a crucial matter in older people's care. Many patients wished to remain in their homes even when they were incapable of looking after themselves. The nurses connected with the need of human beings to want to be self-caring.

The nurses often made ethical decisions regarding home care in the action of giving nursing care, and patients frequently asked for advice. Many close family members felt worried, guilty or anxious and the nurses spent time informing and advising about options, giving 'on the spot' counselling and advice for the relatives. This, of course, has very powerful consequences, not least for the patient who was making decisions concerning where they would choose to live for their remaining life. The nurses gave freely of their time without any restraints of formal appointments or official clinics; in fact, they were a constant source of professional support and advice.

We have to get to a personal level with the patients and their families to find out what the problems are. This will also involve discussing the social outlet as well they tell you all sorts of personal things.

Relatives often expressed feelings of guilt or of not being able to cope. The nurses would always listen and offer advice. The nurses demonstrated that they were learning effectively from their experiences of working with the families. It was noticeable that the decisions made at these times were made on the basis of past experiences. Thus it was the case that the experiences of the nurses were not occurring in isolation from what had happened before but were an accumulation of their past experiences in similar situations, the effect being that each new experience was a mixture of their past and present nursing experiences. This 'stored knowledge' would possibly guide the nurses' practice in the future.

Responding: nurses making judgement in action at the bedside

Responding as a factor was closely linked to the nurses' ability to assess the patient whilst giving care and to respond instantly to a changing situation. The nurses were making decisions concerning patients during the process of giving care.

The nurses constantly assessed their patients' condition by a process of judgement in action, and were critically thinking whilst giving nursing care. It seems that nursing practice does not remain static but is a constant ongoing process of responsiveness on behalf of the nurse. Critical thinking in nursing practice was an active process as the nurses were confronted by patients' activities. This required a degree of creativity. Critical thinking on behalf of the nurses formed a reasoned cycle of action in terms of giving the nursing care there and then. Nursing care changes at a rapid rate dependent upon a patient's needs, condition, progress or deterioration.

'She cannot get around the house independently and I do not think that her husband will manage. I think they may both have to go into a nursing home.' The patient realises that things are getting difficult ... the nurse sits and talks to the patient there and then about the home care.

Responding was not only in the form of clinical interventions, such as changing the patient's position or giving care to the patient's pressure areas to prevent any possible skin breakdown, but also took the form of talking and discussing details of care. Reflection 'in action' and 'on action' was demonstrated at the bedside and it was noted that the nurses were constantly thinking about and acting on the health needs of their patients. In this stance nursing is action oriented.

Nurses were responsive to patients' needs and their decision making and judgements were visible as they actually gave nursing care. Assessment seemed to be completed in action, and through a process of reflection in action the nurses would make conscious decisions about nursing care. If required, these action plans would be implemented there and then. In effect, the nursing documentation lags behind practice, which is an active process.

Judgement in action was important to the nurses' practice. Given the importance of the completion of care plans and the use of nursing models, they were not used to any greater extent as a source of information, with the exception of the handover report between shifts. Whilst the nurses discussed the requirements of having to complete this documentation, the documents themselves did not reflect the in-depth critical thinking which was demonstrated by making judgements in the practice of nursing. This was reflected in Schon's (1990) ideas of the limits of Technical Rationality, which is a positivist epistemology and relies on the assumption that empirical science based on facts and observable features is the only source of knowledge. Indeed, it is this idea that has governed the hierarchical structures of nursing.

The nurses also seemed to be under pressure in the writing of care plans and the use of a nursing model. This was seen to be good nursing practice by their managers. There seemed to be an understanding that these documents were a requirement by managers to show that they had done the work required of them. This was reflected in the fact that the nurses were aware that the nursing documentation was legally required. The technical evidence of the use of the nursing model of Roper et al. (1983) was identified in practice for the gathering of information and was used as a checklist for the nursing formal assessment. Information pertaining to the patient's activities of daily living was obtained at the start of the patient's admission to hospital. Comments by the nurses indicated that the writing up of care plans demonstrated the nursing care that had been delivered, and they were completing one episode of care in order to move onto the next.

Whilst the nurses discussed all the reasons why they should use the models and documentation, they also accepted that they 'ought to use' the nursing models and thought it would be of benefit to their standard of nursing care. However, there seemed to be a difference here in what the nurses 'ought to do' and what they 'actually practised'.

These differences could have been differences between the nurses' espoused theories about the use of nursing models in terms of what they said and the actual theories in use in their daily practice. 'Espoused theory' was the rationale for the use of nursing models. Despite this, the nurses' 'theories in action' were the judgements made by critical thinking processes in action by themselves.

Are you comfortable?

The factor labelled 'comforting' was identified within many themes. Indeed, comfort needs formed a major aspect of the nurses' work. But it was an everyday activity and not regarded by the nurses as a complex issue.

'Are you comfortable?' was a question often asked and nursing the older person was essentially about the comfort need of the patients. Ensuring comfort was seen as a major part of the nurses' work but also an everyday activity that was not described as complex, although it appeared to contain many activities and different forms. The nurses developed awareness and were able to understand when their patients were uncomfortable. Comfort was not an issue that the nurses found difficult and it was a part of all aspects of their work. They sometimes described comfort as an aspect of 'total patient care', which was a term used in the everyday language of the nurses.

Nurses linked the ways that they organised nursing care and this was directly associated with the patients' need for comfort. The nurse–patient relationship was seen as comforting and supporting. This was linked to individual nursing where the nurses were able to get to know the patient and their family, supporting them physically and emotionally. Comfort was linked to the notion of support and love.

In the nursing literature a variety of explanations are given for comfort. In theoretical discussions comfort has been linked to meeting patients' needs. Despite the efforts of theorists, it appears that academics are only beginning to uncover the multidimensional complexity of comfort and how it is achieved. Comfort is a central concept in nursing; however, its contextual meaning in the literature is vague since there are many meanings of the term, some of which can apply in a given situation whilst others are not so applicable. In addition, 'comfort' is frequently used in descriptions relating to the art of nursing.

Morse et al. (1994) suggest that adequate descriptions of comfort have not been clearly developed in research. Using qualitative approaches researchers have attempted to understand the experiences of patients and the ways that comfort is achieved (Morse, 1993).

The author noted that literature pertinent to comfort of the older patient was not easily available. In contrast, the advanced academic literature tended to have highly theoretical accounts of comfort, which were in themselves complex and difficult to operationalise. As Smith (1992) noted, nurses experienced in working in older people's nursing talk positively about their work. Elements of nursing care such as comfort, described by Smith, are difficult to capture and may happen unnoticed in the everyday practice of nursing. If these little things make such a vast improvement to patients' restoration to health, they should not be regarded as superficial by nurses in practice and undocumented by nurse academics. Interestingly, in terms of the theoretical accounts of such care there is a definite lack of documentation about such interventions involving the comfort needs of patients, with a lack of a formal language to describe the work of nurses, because rather bland statements like 'total patient care' and 'tender loving care' were used by the nurses themselves. This was seen as a language of practice in older people's care.

Meyers (2000) suggests there are barriers to the uptake of the findings of traditional research, and suggests using action research which is particularly suited to identifying problems in clinical practice. Action research typically draws on qualitative methods such as interviews and observations. This then could be a way to develop such concepts and to define aspects of comfort.

Ensuring comfort was a major part of the nurses' work and an everyday activity not identified by the nurses as complex. It appeared to contain many activities and different forms. Comfort was referred to when cleaning the mouth, bed bathing or generally attending to the patient.

Collaborating with all multidisciplinary and interagency staff

Effective communication and teamwork was seen as essential for effective patient care. The nature of older people's nursing is difficult and complex and it seemed that the various disciplines could not work in isolation. The multidisciplinary team worked well and had established good communication skills. All members seemed to respect each other's expertise. This is shown in the following examples:

> We did a home assessment with the occupational therapist a few days ago to see the home conditions, and how the patient will manage when he is discharged home.

> She has been in hospital for about a week now so it is a bit early to think about a nursing home, but we will have a multidisciplinary case conference to discuss all possibilities for this patient.

The team approach to nursing care required co-ordination and organisation in order that the responsibility of each member was ensured. The multidisciplinary team had a variety of members with different philosophies of care and traditionally different levels of status and power. This affected the ways in which the team was perceived and acted.

There is a traditional belief that medical staff control practice, which was evident. This medical model essentially had a concentration on physical cure. The doctor appeared to be the head of the team at formal meetings such as case conferences and ward rounds, with other members reporting to the doctors about aspects of a patient's needs. Despite these professional boundaries, it was evident that there was mutual trust and understanding of each other's responsibilities, strengths and constraints.

Therapeutic aspects of care of older people

Hygiene care

Hygiene care included oral hygiene, bed bathing and grooming, all of which were accompanied by a constant ongoing dialogue between nurses and patients. These verbal and non-verbal interactions were significant as they involved the nurses making a constant nursing assessment of the patient's condition. The nurses delivered very personalised care for their patients and were able to talk about the smallest detail of personal information.

We wash, dress and set her hair as well and she likes make-up in the morning. She has her own teeth and we have a very soft toothbrush to clean her teeth. She loves to suck the toothbrush and the family brought in flavoured tooth gel for her lips strawberry is her favourite. We stimulated her senses and the family have brought in L'Aimant perfume as it's her favourite smell. When she has a bed bath we make sure that the patient herself feels clean and she likes hand cream and her nails cleaned. We always have high standards of hygiene. We use her own soaps and perfumes. We use body lotions and peppermint cream for her toes and feet.

The author noted that literature pertinent to hygiene of the older person was not easily available. Most texts on hygiene refer to basic nursing care and are in the main written in the format of procedure manuals (e.g. Royal Marsden Hospital, 2004). These outline how to perform various nursing procedures such as oral hygiene, including the related equipment. In contrast, the advanced academic literature tends to have highly theoretical accounts.

The nurses identified many difficulties that can occur within one episode of hygiene care. When the author read the nursing literature it was often presented as though hygiene as an intervention occurs one at a time, which is not the case. This represents an attempt in the literature to make nursing practice more manageable in terms of academic writing. Nevertheless, in practice patients' problems occur at the same time and become difficult to manage. This issue supports the work of Schon (1990), who suggested that practitioners have to deal with whole problems rather than individual elements. It could also be in the domain of tacit knowledge as described by Polanyi (1956), inasmuch as the skilled practitioner is often unable to give reasons for certain actions or able to state their presuppositions. Additionally, if reasons are given they sometimes sound quite unconvincing. The nurses often referred to the issue of hygiene as 'total patient care', which was a generalised way of describing specific aspects of nursing care.

It seems that nurses are using different kinds of knowledge in their practice. In particular they use 'know how' knowledge, demonstrated in their practical expertise and skill. However, Benner (1984) suggested that it is the practical knowledge such as this that has not been adequately described. Nurses were able to give a scientific account of the prevention of dehydration and infection and referred to knowledge of physiology, bacteriology and pharmacology as formal sources of knowledge learned in nurse education.

Nurses referred specifically to their nurse education as a significant influence on how they performed their nursing care and valued the knowledge learned. They indicated that this was thought of as a form of authoritative knowledge. Benner (1984) suggested that nurses have common meanings in practice that are developed over time and shared, as in the illustrations above. The care of a highly dependent patient on bed rest is known by nurses as requiring a high nursing input involving the prevention of the hazards of bed rest (Carroll, 1993). However, the therapeutic interventions that address hygiene requirements are usually documented in a fairly superficial way and each issue is often dealt with separately through a concept clarification framework.

Elimination care

A large amount of time was spent by the nurses on elimination care, with the nurses often having to develop a care plan to meet the individual needs of patients. The nurses regarded continence as an important factor in terms of the patient's dignity (DoH, 2006).

The problems associated with urinary and faecal incontinence were an aspect of nursing care related to the patient's self-esteem and dignity, as well as the obvious problems of hygiene, skin care and other physical problems. The issue was regarded as important in that the nurses kept records in the care plans of the patients' elimination needs. This was identified in the Roper et al. nursing model (1983) as an essential daily activity.

This issue shows the way in which nurses constantly encourage immobile older patients to care for themselves, and the level of detail necessary in even an apparently simple movement. Patients asked the nurse for a bedpan or to go to the toilet. Some nurses would spend time talking, encouraging and explaining that it would be good exercise for the patients to see if they could manage to walk. Often the nurse would link this to getting ready to go home. This reminder of going home was seen as a particular type of encouragement that clearly had significant benefits for motivating the patient.

The author reviewed many nursing textbooks and much literature on older people's nursing to compare nursing episodes with the academic literature on that subject, and to see whether the nurses' actions were the same as that advocated within the theoretical literature. An example of this is the notion of encouragement during mobilising and rehabilitation as an important issue for discussion and recommendation. However, only small sections were found, and sometimes a few lines briefly mentioning this. This, then, could be a personal paradigm case as described by Rolfe et al. (2001), where practitioners have their own directory or chunks of solutions to particular events. The issue of encouragement is an example where professional understanding and experience does not emanate from the theoretical literature but rather derives from a cumulative body of personal knowledge gained from the nurses' experiences of different older people's care in a nursing situation.

The patient has come into the unit for rehabilitation prior to being discharged home. He has been admitted for assessment, but he is very reluctant to move and would like to stay in bed all day. It's important to encourage him to be as mobile as possible and we start gently by walking him back and forth to the toilet. Sometimes he will just walk to the toilet and we will bring him back in the wheelchair. We take things slowly.

A nurse recognised that the patient was reluctant to walk to the toilet and was becoming dependent on the nurses. This assessment was made on the perceptual understanding of the person and their normal routine. The concept of knowing the person seemed to have influenced how the nurse organised her care. Distinctions such as this are an example of judgements in action. This practical knowledge depends on the nurse knowing her patient as a person and being familiar with the patient's response patterns.

Nutritional care

The nurses frequently assessed nutritional needs, where there were many difficult issues. These were dealt with by the staff together with the involvement of the family.

The dietician has been counselling the husband about diabetes and his wife's nutrition generally. She will only allow her husband to do most for her. She does respond to us when she wants to though.

The patients' relatives were encouraged to help with feeding. As Benner (1984) noted, professional artistry involves much more than applying the body of knowledge; it requires the cognitive skills to use knowledge critically and creatively, plus a high level of self-awareness and the ability to see the uniqueness of each clinical situation in order to learn from those experiences. By working with the family, the nurses were able to achieve aspects of nursing care that they found difficult, such as a frail patient refusing to eat.

The nurses continually had to deal with difficult problems associated with nutrition and patient compliance, often relying on the family to be involved in the care. The development of emotional closeness between the nurse and patient allowed opportunities for therapeutic intervention to develop.

A theme of nutrition emerged, which contained many issues relating to helping patients with fluids or feeding. The nurses often worked with the relatives to assist with feeding. There were aspects referring to the nurse advising the patient about their nutrition and special diets. There were also difficult situations noted in practice. The following are examples:

> The patient's feeds are performed via the gastrostomy tube, he does have problems of loose bowel actions from time to time with this method of feed.

> She will only eat food that her husband brings in and will close her mouth and refuse to eat for the nurses.

Medication and pain control

Pain control was a theme linked to the comfort needs of the patient. Argyris and Schon (1974), discussing theories of action, described examples when a practitioner knows in a certain situation what to do.

> The patient was now complaining of pain in her leg, which was gangrenous. The nurse looked at the treatment chart and commented that the patient had already received analgesic from the night staff, and was not due for further analgesia. The nurse talked to the patient and comforted her by offering small sips of water, from the beaker, a fan was switched on as cool comfort and the nurse telephoned the doctor.

The nurse in this example recognised that the pain level was increasing above the level of the prescribed analgesia and the consequence was that the patient was becoming restless. The nurse responded immediately with the appropriate actions in the situation by offering comforting measures and by asking the doctor on call to visit the ward immediately and examine the patient.

The nurse's management of the patient's pain assessment included assumptions about herself as an advocate for the patient, the wellbeing and safety of the patient, the individual situation and the connections of her actions and the doctor by advising him to see the patient immediately. The nurse was demonstrating an awareness of the consequences of the patient's pain levels in that given situation. The pattern of the practice theory was:

the nurse felt a sense of responsibility;
safety factors were a priority;
the individual context of the situation was considered;
the nurse identified the connections between all the factors, which were pain, accountability, safety, responsibility.

This action is clearly in the domain of 'know how' knowledge, sometimes described as the art of nursing. 'Know how' knowledge is acquired through practice and experience. There was also evidence of propositional knowledge in the nurse's understanding of the pharmacology of pain relief and the use of a cooling fan on a painful extremity.

Schon, discussing expert practitioners, suggested that an expert draws on his or her experiences and selects an approach based on a wide range of paradigms in practice. This was different from following a hospital procedure, which would be planned in advance in a prescriptive way. The nurse's knowing was in action.

Professional skill, as discussed by Benner (1984), does not always come from advanced theoretical knowledge but may develop from the nurse's personal knowledge of similar situations. From the above statement, the nurse has developed the ability to recognise a situation where the patient needed relief and reassurance, and would have had a range of alternative strategies that could have been implemented if necessary. This was reiterated by Boud et al. (1985), who identified a process of reflective evaluation and who suggested that practitioners learn by making connections between events, a process they refer to as association. This enables the nurse to learn effectively from experience and it is necessary to establish connections between events that occur.

The nurses often worked with the relatives to assist with feeding. There were statements referring to the nurse advising the patient about their nutrition and special diets. There were also difficult situations noted in practice.

Preventative and safety issues

Many of the nurses referred to patients' safety when talking about the clinical aspects of their work – when performing aseptic dressing techniques, for example. They were constantly theorising in action and able to give a good rationale about the potential problems. They were aware of the fact that an older patient might fall or collapse unexpectedly and demonstrated a personal working theory on potential hazards.

Nurses referred to the need to assess their patients' level of dependency and were constantly working towards preparing patients for discharge home and getting them as mobile as possible. One of the main issues discussed was the question of how safe an older person was to live alone on discharge. Although mobilising patients is seen as a central issue in patient care, it became evident that this therapeutic intervention was so much a part of all aspects of care it was sometimes difficult to identify it as a separate therapy. It could also be misinterpreted as basic care. In addition, theoretical accounts about aspects of mobility tend to focus on the physiological and functional aspects of motor skills. The literature referring to mobility refers to the work of other members of the multidisciplinary team and seems to suggest that mobility is the remit of the physiotherapist. However, in practice it was an essential remit of the nursing staff.

Difficult problems are encountered on a daily basis. Some of these are major issues that not only affect the patient's care in hospital but also the difficulty of the carers being able to manage when the patient is discharged home. These crucial issues have to be resolved. The author observed several episodes where nursing interventions such as these would be discussed by the patient and nurse. The nurses always allowed time for discussions and constantly encouraged patients to make their own choices. A safety theme developed which contained aspects of nursing care referring to safety issues.

I was able to give suction to the patient, as her breathing was bubbly prior to the occupational therapist working with her. This made the patient more comfortable and maintained a clear airway.

Issues relating to the control of cross-infection were referring to aseptic technique, pressure area care and hand washing. There was an understanding demonstrated by the nurses concerning the transmission, prevention and containment of infection.

The author was aware that issues relating to preventative issues contained actions that demonstrated that the nurses were constantly striving to prevent problems of immobility in their patients. They wanted to prevent patients from becoming bed-bound and there were constant comments regarding the safety of the patient when walking alone. This was linked to issues of rehabilitation and preparing the patient to be self-caring when returning home. Rehabilitation was seen as the process by which patients were helped back to being as well as they could be. This involved teaching them to regain lost skills and thus to regain independence.

Safety issues were considered extremely important by the nurses and this was reflected in the large number of statements on this theme.

Collegial interactions

Documented empirical evidence suggests that sometimes nurses are not perceived as making a major contribution to the rehabilitative process and are not viewed as the driving force within the process. Terms such as 'maintaining' and 'caring' are frequently used in describing the nurse's role. Such literature suggests that nurses are seen to have a secondary rather than primary function in rehabilitation. However, the nurses in this study clearly demonstrated an ability to work within a team, carrying an advisory and a lead role. They were involved and took the lead in discussions with therapists to make decisions on the best way forward with a patient's care. The team approach required co-ordination in order that the responsibility of each member of the team was ensured. In the everyday working practice of older people's nursing care there were examples of theorising in action in a team approach.

Nursing assessment

It is widely recognised that the medical problems associated with the care of older people are multidimensional since the patient often has more than one medical and nursing issue (Reed and Robbins, 1991; Iliffe and Drennan, 2003; Nolan et al., 2004; McCormack and McCance, 2006).

Older patients are often afflicted with numerous health problems that require specialised nursing assessment. The nurses discussed ageing as a factor in the assessment process and demonstrated an in-depth theoretical knowledge of this. In addition, acute problems may develop, the onset often being detected by the nurse monitoring the patient's progress. It would appear that older patients, as well as their care givers, may ignore potential medical difficulties; they are often dismissive of problems associated with poor habits such as eating incorrectly, putting them down to old age. Also, patients frequently take numerous medications that may mask or confuse symptoms of disease or may even themselves be the cause of the problems. The nurses were able to discuss patients' medical problems and relate these to the problems encountered by the patients and their carers.

Caring and supporting the older person and their carers

Nursing care is regularly described in such well-known phrases as 'total patient care' and 'holistic nursing care'. The words 'care' and 'caring' are embodied in the everyday language of nursing and caring has been widely portrayed as important to nursing.

Issues such as patients not being able to cope at home or having to make a decision to move to a nursing home were sometimes discussed during interventions. It may be the case that at these very private times the patient felt close to the nurse. Often the nurse's communication skills were extremely advanced. The nurse would sit and hold the patient's hand, taking time to support and encourage him or her to make choices. It was during these times the patient would often discuss very personal issues and disclose their anxieties and fears, such as the loss of their loved one. Nursing older people was not just about physical care; it also involved a close working relationship and companionship.

The demonstration of concern has been linked significantly to caring, inasmuch as what the patient is experiencing is important to the nurse as a person. To work with a patient must involve the nurse being concerned for that patient. Concern also encompasses empathy, where one attempts to view the world as the other person experiences it and communicate this knowing to the patient. Although caring is a loosely defined concept, many theorists recognise a distinction between caring about and caring for someone. In general terms, to care about someone suggests an attachment or an emotional relationship but does not distinguish necessarily the practical activities or giving time to that person. Additionally, from a sociological stance this comparison between caring about and caring for has been associated with informal and formal aspects of care. Caring about is identified with unpaid care, emotional involvement and the private domain, while caring for is linked with paid work and the public domain. In terms of nursing, the meaning of older people's nursing can appear to fall between caring for and caring about. Empirical nursing studies support this notion. Smith et al. (2003) included a process of being emotionally present, noting that although there may be a sharing of feelings, what distinguishes this form of caring from others is that the nurse cares without obliging the patient to follow in the same way. There is no expectation of reciprocity. Moreover, such giving of self may be evident in the way that the nurse presents herself to the patient and this presence may have an effect on the patient's wellbeing.

Communication, love and companionship

The nurses viewed nursing as a holistic process in which the nurse engaged with the family to foster growth and learning and to deliver nursing care.

> *The patient needs 'total nursing care' she had a brother living in the area and daughter. The family is totally supporting of each other. Her sister read to the patient from the beginning and spoke to her, and we have developed a means of communication with the patient.*

The nurse in this case demonstrated practice knowledge of communication and, although unable to communicate directly with the patient, developed an ability to gather facts by communicating with the family to collect detailed information about her. Working in this way with the relatives, the respondent demonstrated concern for their wellbeing by talking and being with them.

These examples from the practice of care of older people show how the nurse–patient relationship appeared to have been of benefit to the patient, family and the development of the nurse. The closeness displayed in these nursing episodes achieved outcomes of a therapeutic nurse and patient relationship. The nurses regarded the family and the individual patient's personal profile as being significant in the care and through this emerged a unique nurse–patient relationship. The individual communication skills required were identified in practical situations. The nurse demonstrated her ability by utilising her knowledge of communication and adapting this in an individual way within the patient's care. The evidence showed that the nurse was able to identify with the patient at an individual level.

The way in which the nurses perceived the notion of love and companionship was broadly similar. They demonstrated the ability to develop a good rapport and spoke of good communication as being essential. It is interesting that many of the nurses referred to their work as 'good basic care'. Communication was viewed as the essence of companionship between the nurses and their patients. Even when a patient was unable to talk, the nursing staff were often able to find ways of communicating.

Often nurses would refer to 'being close' to their patients, which implied that the nurse felt at ease with the patient. This related to a mutual acceptance of a relationship in which it was possible for the patient to talk freely without embarrassment. Some nurses referred to 'being there' for their patients, suggesting that nurses may sometimes be the only people that the older patients feel able to talk to about such things as loss, grief, loneliness and bereavement.

Accountability and autonomy

Issues concerning accountability and autonomy were discussed as part of the nurses' working patterns. Many of the nurses talked about being in charge and being a constant source of advice to patients, family and colleagues in the multidisciplinary team. The nature of older people's care is such that the nurses felt a sense of responsibility because they were constantly dealing with vulnerable patients who were sometimes mentally confused. The nurses felt that primary nursing allowed them to be more accountable for their patients. Being the named nurse allowed them to get to know and feel closer to the patients and their families.

However, change and development may result from research which gives new approaches to practice. In this study, the nurse had advanced her practice working as a named nurse and was able to perform advanced clinical skills but was restrained by the policies of the management system. It is interesting to note the relationship between knowledge and power. Although the nurse had the knowledge to act, her managers did not give her the power. Accountability was linked to professionalism but was also associated with responsibility and authority. However, in practice accountability and authority both required a sound knowledge base for practice and also the support and authority to act.

Difficult decisions were discussed when the more personal level of care was being delivered. This was an interesting phenomenon, as the literature on information giving suggests a more formal interviewing process. It seems that the bond or trusting relationship built up between the nurses and their patients enhanced a professional closeness. The patients would often disclose their worst fears and the nurses would have to advise them.

The nurses seemed to feel that they were able to represent the best interests of their patients. There were comments showing that nurses explained medical care to patients following the doctors' rounds. The nurses would explain a procedure to the patient if they did not understand the original explanation given by the medical staff. This reflected the importance of the advocate role of the nurses.

There was also evidence that occasionally the nurses seemed to be prevented from developing their practice because of the management system. This was interesting given the fact that these nurses were more autonomous in their nursing practice through primary nursing. Yet, despite this, they did not always have the authority to act. It was surprising that the nurses, although they had been given more authority to act autonomously as accountable professionals, still had to convince both the medical profession and their managers that they could be trusted with that authority.

The nurses were making decisions about patients' future home arrangements. They said these were extremely difficult decisions to handle in practice. This was because it raised ethical dilemmas for them about helping the patients and their families make the correct decisions. Sometimes the nurses said that patients often wanted to go back to live in their own homes when they were in fact incapable of maintaining their own safety. There was sometimes a risk of falling and safety was naturally seen as a major issue. Redfern (2006) discusses multidisciplinary assessment, and advocates that no one individual health or social or healthcare worker will have the skills and knowledge to undertake home assessments alone. A variety of assessment strategies may be necessary to capture as comprehensive picture as possible.

The patient had deteriorated since the death of her husband. She was admitted to this ward after having falls at home, and safety is a major issue here.

Named nursing was described as a professional model of practice in which the qualified nurses were responsible and accountable for the nursing care, during the entire duration of their stay, of a case-load of patients. The advantage of named nursing was that it enabled the nurses to establish better relationships and communicate more easily with patients and their relatives.

The patient is in a nursing bed, which means that I am the key person responsible for arranging the patient care. I call the GP if there is any medical intervention needed, but really the patient is a nursing issue.

Assessment of the home and family care

The use of critical thinking skills was evident during episodes of nursing care, particularly in relation to the assessment of the home and family situation. There was evidence of clinical reasoning, with consideration being given to the individualised physical and affective outcomes, and this affected the perceptions of the nursing focus. The nurses had to make judgements there and then, with thoughtful activities pertaining to what was the best decision for the patient's nursing care. The nurses had to continuously review and transform their understandings and consider alternatives. Critical thinking was seen as reasoning with a view to creating effective nursing outcomes.

I usually do the dressings to the gangrenous ulcer about half an hour after the medication to ensure that the patient is more comfortable and pain free. Although it is difficult to manage her as she is so frail.

The process of risk assessment seemed to be embedded in many aspects of the nurses' work with the older patients. The more involved in the assessment they became the more it was evident that there was an area of intuitive understanding in their decision making about the assessment of risk. Some of the nurses seemed able to make particularly sensitive judgements about whether the patient was unstable or unsafe to walk alone. It is often easy to forget the complex nature of learning, practice experience and supervision required, which comes from experience of specialist nursing practice and underpins this assessment process.

Risk assessment was often seen as identifying potential problems in nursing care: issues relating to physical risks such as falling, social care risks or being unable to look after themselves in the future.

The nurse helps the patient into the toilet, and instructs the patient to hold onto the handrail as the nurse said there was always the risk of him having further falls. The patient shuffles around with the respondent constantly supporting his balance.

Carers and relatives

The nurses spent a great deal of time in building a relationship with the patients' families, and this was seen as important in making a comprehensive assessment of the home and availability of future family care. Building a relationship was about negotiation, and the views of the families were seen as crucial. Smith et al. (2003) suggest that there is a willingness of the family and carers to become more engaged with looking after their elders, but they require more information and advice.

The involvement of the carers and relatives in patient care was viewed as good nursing practice. The family appeared to be a major factor in the patients' progress. Some nurses indicated that if the family received support they were more able to contribute to the patients' management in the future. Greater involvement of relatives also facilitated a closer relationship between nurse and relative with improved communication.

Clearly, nursing is an active process which requires constant problem solving and the utilising of critical thinking skills and understanding in a practice situation. This involves reflection in action and on action. Nurses discussed the ward using the Roper, Logan and Tierney (1983) model of nursing to assess the patients. In British nursing there seems to be a wide acceptance of nursing models generally and particularly of Roper et al. However, the nurses tended to use the nursing model documentation as a checklist only, filling in the forms and using the documents in a rigid way. Nurses indicated that it was often difficult to know in which box to record information, as it did not appear on the activities of daily living. Nursing issues seemed to be dealt with in action through a working knowledge of the patients.

Reed and Robbins (1991) suggested that nursing models were used as a starting point for the development of nursing theory. However, the adoption of nursing models has become widespread in nursing with little empirical evidence to support their use and little evidence of critical evaluation. There seems to have been a lack of strategy in the initial introduction of nursing models. This has now led to nurses using documents that they do not understand or value (Smith, 2003).

The nurses were constantly concerned with risk assessment. They would often work in pairs to assist each other if they felt there was a risk in managing the patients on their own. Some nurses spoke about the risk of lifting the patients and used mechanical hoists whenever possible, although sometimes the patients were too frail. Clearly the nurses needed to manage the risk situation there and then. They also had to work within the multidisciplinary team to assess the risks of the future care of the older person.

In a way that is the advantage of being the named nurse as I am able to constantly assess the patient on a daily basis and also provide continuity for her daughter. We have to care for the family in older people's care, which includes assessing how the carers are coping as well.

Difficult decisions are disclosed to the nurses about whether or not the older patient could be managed by their family after discharge. The nurses would allow time to talk, to discuss and explain to the older person about the decision.

Empirical evidence suggests that generally the hospital discharge of patients is handled poorly, and the Royal College of Nursing issued a series of research-based recommendations on hospital discharge directed at managers and policy makers. However, the nurses themselves worked by assessing the patient's ability on a daily basis and by working together with the multidisciplinary team and planning, with the family, the way forward. There were clearly many issues that were extremely difficult in practice and these would be discussed in a case conference by the whole team. Rather like a jigsaw puzzle, each piece of information from each member of the team would be shared and pieced together until the whole problem emerged. From this close collaboration, decisions were reached and implemented.

The nurses were involved with the families of the older patients and encouraged the family to be involved in the nursing care. All the wards observed had an open visiting policy, a very important matter for older relatives, who may be living in rural areas and do not want to be restricted to evening visiting. Assessment was visible in the actions of the nurses whilst giving nursing care. It was evident that the nurses needed to respond and assess problems there and then, sometimes dealing with more than one issue in each episode of care.

Person-centred framework

McCormack and McCance (2006) advocate a person-centred framework and the care environment construct focuses on the context in which care is delivered – systems that allow shared decision making, effective staff relationships. McCormack also proposes person-centred processes which focus on delivering care through a range of activities, which include working with patients' beliefs and values, having a sympathetic presence, sharing decision making and providing physical needs. This framework, which is a mid-range theory, has implications for understanding the practice of nursing older people. The person-centred framework discussed the complexity of the dimensions of humanistic caring practice and McCormack encourages nurses to move beyond the focus on technical skills and nurses to engage in this type of practice. McCormack embraces all forms of knowing and acting to promote choice and partnership in care decision making.

The research presented in this book shows the value of going into practice and, by observing and interviewing nurses, has shown that nurses were working in an individual and person-centred way. This was similar to McCormack's framework (described above) and addresses the changing perspectives of caring for older people with the advent of person-centred care and relationship-centred care (Nolan, 2004).

Conclusion

This chapter has shown the practical ways in which nurses solved problems in practice that occurred every day when they gave direct nursing care. The factors of practice theory were embedded within their personal framework and were shown to be the source of care for older people.

Chapter 6 will focus on the practice of caring for older people.

Suggested reading

Benner, P. (1984) *From Novice to Expert: Excellence and Power in Clinical Nursing Practice* (Menlo Park, CA: Addison-Wesley). This is a research book based on the skills performance in the development of an expert nurse. Issues considered are competencies, advanced beginners, change processes, and case studies as exemplars.

Drake, R. F. (2001) *The Principles of Social Policy* (Basingstoke: Palgrave Macmillan). This book looks at social policy as shaped by prevailing political beliefs and values, made tangible in the form of overarching policy objectives.

Hill, M. (2003) *Understanding Social Policy*, 7th edition (Malden, MA: Blackwell Publishing). This book considers policy innovations. It looks at new policy linkages between social security and employment, child care and education. There is a new section regarding social divisions.

Kane, R. L. and Kane, R. A. (2000) *Assessing Older Persons: Measures, Meaning and Practical Applications* (Oxford: Oxford University Press). This book looks at assessment, function, health, emotion, cognition and social wellbeing. It also discusses family care givers, physical environments, preferences, spirituality and satisfaction. It looks critically at various assessment tools.

Redfern, S. and Ross, M. (2006) *Nursing Older People*, 4th edition (London: Churchill Livingstone). This textbook provides supporting literature to care of older people. The 4th edition contains major policy initiatives and organisational changes in health and social care.

Focusing on the practice of caring for older people

This chapter:

▶ explores ways to develop practice theory directly from nursing care of older people;
▶ identifies a family of practice for older people's nursing care;
▶ discusses the uniqueness of individual practice.

Developing practice theory from care of older people

The framework presented in Chapter 5 raises an interesting question regarding the development of the knowledge of nursing directly from the practice of nursing. Theories of older people's nursing are built up inductively from nursing practice itself. Inductive research of the kind being discussed, which consider the informal theory cycle in practice, can be found in Lincoln and Guba (1985) and Denzin and Lincoln (2005).

In an era of evidence-based practice, research from a positivist standpoint does have a place, and always has done. For example, the arguments in editorials of qualitative research journals tend to revolve around how qualitative research provides answers to different questions and so has a place in its own right. The use of qualitative research is seen as a way of developing practice by asking questions relevant to older people, their families and staff who care for them. There does remain a place for large-scale studies that measure outcomes for older people. Nurses should be given the skills of critical appraisal to enable them to access relevant research that is relevant to their practice.

Theory generation about care of older people

The traditional scientific positivist research could sometimes be inadequate for theory generation in a practice-based discipline of nursing. This is because each nursing situation is about individual people and practice (Eraut, 1994; Nolan et al., 2004; McCormack, 2004). Inductive theory building from practice is context specific, relating to particular situations in practice. Formal theory is different as it relates to global situations and exists independently of practice.

The technical rationality model assumes that theoretical knowledge must be the foundation of practice because it is research-generated, systematic and scientific. It is a knowledge that takes the form of generalised propositions. Furthermore, the 'worthwhileness' of theoretical knowledge is reinforced because of the apparent ability of theoretical knowledge to make predictions about events. As Usher et al. point out, 'the way that technical-rationality constitutes the relationship between theory and practice is strongly contested. There is a much greater readiness to reject the notion that theoretical knowledge can simply be applied or mapped onto practice' (1997: 126). Schon (1990) reminds us that knowledge is performative rather than propositional and that practice is centred on action. Moreover, as discussed, practice was about a particular kind of action, as it was neither random behaviour nor was it behaviour predictable from a body of theoretical knowledge. Rather, it was appropriate – or the right – action depending on the context and situation of each nursing episode for each older patient.

Scientific nursing

Nurses were able to identify and use large-scale studies and give scientific accounts of the practice. They talked about bacteriology, pharmacology and physiology as formal sources of knowledge learned in nurse education courses. They referred to their nurse education as a significant influence on how they performed their nursing care, and valued the knowledge they had gained in clinical placements.

Redfern and Ross's (2006) book *Nursing Older People* provides a very comprehensive textbook on nursing older people. Its approach and content is relevant to practitioners from all disciplines. It gives detailed knowledge needed to care for older people, and focuses on evidence-based care and the effectiveness of interventions that support older people.

Pause for thought

Can you think of a situation in your own practice where you had to think on your feet? Did the textbook theory on that situation give you all the answers you required?

In the study, in terms of the technical interventions, there was a substantial amount of empirical evidence to support what the nurses did in their practice. Therefore, the scientific knowledge within the nursing literature supported practice. However, the nurses had to respond to difficult situations quickly and often there were no easy answers. Some nurses discussed their experiences in practice and felt this was important.

Theory and practice of care of older people

Experiential knowledge, then, seemed to arise from practice. In unique situations practitioners have to draw on their experience and select an approach based on a wide range of issues in practice. They then have to synthesise this information and apply it when the actions they should take are not clear. The nurses gave personal paradigm care where they had their own repertoire of solutions to particular events. They had developed the ability to interpret a situation and implement an action plan. This is supported by authors such as Eraut (1994), who suggests there are distinctions between formal knowledge and practical know-how, which is inherent in practitioners' actions.

This, then, may be another way of conceptualising the theory–practice gap. The author found there was academic theory and evidence-based research available to explain the technical aspects of nursing such as cross-infection, medication care of pressure sores, and mobility. However, there is little in the way of how to nurse someone in the fullest and broadest sense of the word: how to relieve burdens and fear of the unknown, how to help the patient cope with loss of dignity, and how to encourage their ability to look after themselves.

Advising and monitoring patient care standards

The nurses discussed their role as being a key figure in the overall management of the ward, and talked about continuity of care as a major issue. The nurses were the constant source of information to all staff and visitors and were the only members of the multidisciplinary team constantly within the ward. Nurses stayed with their patients for the duration of their span of duty. This of course gave the nurses every opportunity to be responsible and in charge of patient care. On many occasions nurses would be interrupted by a member of the multidisciplinary team requesting information regarding the patient. This would also happen during the times when nursing care was being administered behind the screens.

Sources of knowledge in care of older people

There is evidence that the nurses had learned about the care they gave formally in their nurse education programmes and valued the teaching received from their nurse lecturers. They had attended post-registration certificate and diploma courses in older people's nursing, teaching and assessing, counselling, and continence promotion. All of these educational courses enabled the trained nurses to utilise textbooks on older people's care, distance learning packs, e-learning modules, journals and research reports.

Nurses read weekly journals such as the *Nursing Times, Nursing Standard* and *Professional Nurse*. Some nurses referred to advanced nursing journals which they perceived as using highly jargonistic academic language. In practice the nurses identified with experiential learning, often referring to their past experiences as a source of knowledge. A mentor system seemed to enhance the learning process, where nurses were constantly seeking advice from a more experienced nurse.

All of the nursing care described shows how the work of nursing in caring for older people is patient centred. The factors of practice theory that were identified were constant elements. These, put together, show that the nursing practice had a framework of practice theory.

Philosophy: a family of practice

The framework described in this book shared the same purposes and goals, in that they were about nursing practice. The factors are a family of practice about individual patients and the need to nurture and rehabilitate older patients. They were not talked about within the literature of older people's nursing.

‎ause for thought

Consider your own practice or a particular episode from nursing care that you have had recently. What was your intention or purpose for the patient? What was the significance of your actions for that person?

The framework: nursing care of a similar kind

The nursing care of older people in the framework shown in this book was about the formal and final causes of caring for older patients (see Croche, 1920). There is a type of family resemblance among the combinations but it is not dependent on a strict identity of all of them. There were characteristics that exist between all members of the family, yet no one family member had all of the exact individual features. They involved the more tangible and complex nature of human interaction and were contextual and individual. The factors identified involved those ingredients or elements that were of a similar kind.

They were practice orientated and very much performed in action by the nurses. Wittgenstein (1967) showed that instances of this nature fall under the example of a family or towards a particular case. The point that Wittgenstein's understanding brings out is that the resemblance between the things to which the same word applies may be of different degrees. The nursing care episodes were similar at varying degrees. Their strongest link was that they were relating to the practice of the nurses caring for older people.

Wittgenstein's philosophy

The framework discussed has similar features, which resembled holistic patient-centred nursing care. The nurses focused their nursing care on the individual needs of their older patients. A patient is seen as a complex individual with a particular range of needs. Wittgenstein's philosophy about classifications, language and their meaning allows alternative ways of interpreting the informal practice theories of older people's nursing.

The author became aware of the complex individual and personal commitments shown by the nurses and the degree to which their own informal practice theories had developed in the nursing practice of caring for older people. There was evidence of informal theorising in action and the use of individual personal theories by the nurses (Box 6.1). This personal reflexivity indicates the close commitment shown by the nurses to the patients. It also illustrates the ways in which the nurses recognised the patient as an individual person with their own needs and personal perspectives and concerns.

Box 6.1   Reflexive notes

Author's reflexivity: What nursing really means
I have become increasingly aware of the diversities of nursing practice in caring for older patients. And I have come to realise the degree to which the nurses' personal identity and their commitment to their patients helped to motivate the patients to want to get better. It seems that for these nurses, nursing older people was not just about doing the procedural clinical aspects of nursing care. The whole of nursing was much more than doing a dressing, or giving an injection. Nursing the older person seems in some way to be about the consideration of the person whom the nurse is caring for, at that time, sharing that person's hopes, worries and sometimes their worst fears. This sharing may help the patient to bear the burden of their ill health and the frustration at their inability to look after themselves.

This raises important points in the development of nursing theories by demonstrating that there are unarticulated nursing theories that are personalised and very much used in the practice of older people's nursing. The informal practice theories also appeared as a family of practice. Empirical propositional theory relating to the clinical experiences cannot capture the know-how of the complicated clinical situations that the nurses were encountering.

In education Carr (1986) suggested that practice is an intentional activity and as such contains its own internal theory. Informal theory of this kind refers to Benner's (1984) know-how and is not something which has been applied to nursing practice, but rather informal theory that is implicit in practice. Usher and Bryant (1997) refer to this as informal theory. Schon (1991) suggested that each practitioner builds up a situational repertoire which is constantly being developed and modified in practice. It seems that nursing theorists have been developing a grand theory of nursing without informal practice theory being acknowledged, uncovered and valued in nursing theory development.

Informal practice theorising within older people's nursing practice

Theoretical literature suggests that the use of nursing models optimises nursing care. This study demonstrated that grand nursing theory is too general to provide much guidance for nurses who have very specific issues of assessment of care of the older person in practice to deal with 'there and then'. McCormack (2003; McCormack and McCance, 2006) suggests that models of nursing, irrespective of their philosophical underpinnings, emphasise the importance of relationships. However, in person-centred nursing, the relationship between nurses and the older person is key to successful nursing care (see Figure 6.1).

Nursing models and theories: do they fit with nursing?

It seems, in nursing generally, there has been a use of nursing models in the United Kingdom. Some nurses indicated that they used nursing models because the nursing management expected them to;

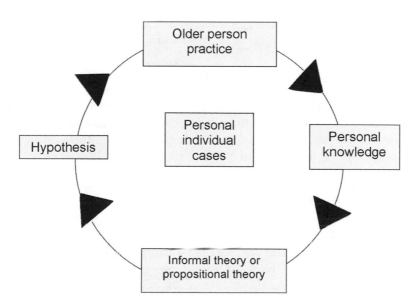

Figure 6.1   Informal practice theorising within older people's nursing practice

and because nobody in authority has told them to stop using nursing models they continue using them.

The nurses tended to complete the documentation by using the activities of daily living as a checklist. This could, however, create an impression that the nurses had not completed the assessment or did not consider certain activities of living important enough. They used the documentation in a stereotyped way that led to the information being collected in a reductionist manner, which may in fact encourage a functional focus to practice. Some nurses indicated that it was often difficult to know in which box to record certain information about the patient, for example, the patient's pain, or bereavement and counselling. These issues were managed by the nurses in practice but the documentation did not mention these. This seems to suggest that the nurses tended to fit the patient to the model rather than use the model to assess the patient. However, they demonstrated a working knowledge of each of their patients. It seems that, above all, the nurses knew the patients as people better than any of the other members of the team:

> *This patient lives alone after suffering the death of her husband two years ago. They were devoted to each other. The patient has deteriorated since and has been admitted for assessment. I have taken time to get to know her who she is and about her life. We have a close relationship now and she tells me all her worries and I share her problems with her and it helps her to cope with her life after the bereavement.*

It is clear that the nurses were continually assessing their patients; they changed the care based on their critical thinking and decision making at the patient's bedside. The nurses spent time recording their decisions after giving the nursing care. This was an interesting feature. It seemed to be the case that they were using their intuitive experiences, as described, to form representations about their individual patients. However, the documentation in no way matched the actions and experiences that the nurses were encountering in their daily practice. The nursing model documentation has been formed by abstract and not action-based theorising, and the nurses used the nursing models in a mechanistic way. The patients' records and nursing notes, including the care plan documents and daily nursing records, were kept in the ward Sister's office. The nurses tended to use the records for formal ward reporting at the shift handover. The records were brought up to date at the end of the morning and afternoon. Views on care planning by the nurses seemed to suggest this:

All the care plans are kept in the office and we update them regularly, although the nursing model does not really reflect the problems that we deal with in care of the older patients. There are no identified problems of older people in Roper's et al. model; after all, the entire model is used in every speciality in nursing. The model is fairly general really. There are specific issues of concern in caring for older patients which we deal with in practice, which are not recognised on the models and documentation.

The nurses did not attach much meaning to the nursing records as being able to represent the nursing care delivered. The documentation lagged behind the actual practice of nursing, which was about the nurses' experiences.

Some nurses were not satisfied with the nursing models or the documentation. They suggested the model was inappropriate because there were problems fitting the patient profile into the model. In addition, there was no mention of the patient's views or of family involvement, this being a major issue in older people's nursing. These, of course, are issues concerning formal and final causes as described by Taylor (1985) (in Benner and Wrubel, 1989: 31): 'Viewing the person as an agent of significance, that is, a being that has concerns and issues.' There seemed to be a mismatch between practice and the documentation in use, which was evident from observation of the practice:

We usually record the care on the care plan and update the record at the end of the morning. It's easier that way. But really all the care is planned when you are with the patient and the family at the bedside, as it were. The forms are very restricted to bodily needs, but caring for older patients is much more holistic and complex. The care plans try to simplify nursing I suppose. It's not that straightforward in practice.

It appeared that the nurses were sometimes expected to utilise nursing models for their care planning. However, in terms of the documentation, this had little impact upon the nursing actions. The theoretical literature suggests that nursing models optimise nursing care. A difference was noted between the theoretical literature on nursing models and the assessment in action in the nursing episodes observed. This identifies that they have not been adequately shaped by nursing practice and are thus under-investigated by nurses themselves.

Pause for thought

Do you use a nursing model in your practice? Reflect on its value and use. What methods do you use to assess older patients?

Clearly, the nursing model in use was not giving direction to practice and not giving assistance to the nurses in understanding the realities of nursing practice. Although grand nursing theories were not intended for use in practice situations, nursing concepts are widely used in current nursing theory development. They have been advocated as providing the 'building blocks' from which theories can be built. Despite this, the theoretical literature usually presents nursing concepts in a singular way. This implies that nursing is intervention led and each intervention occurs one at a time. The complexity of nursing was such that the nurses were dealing with several issues at one time and in doing so demonstrated an ability to assess the patient and to attend to all the needs in action. This is supported by several authors (e.g. Polanyi, 1967; Benner, 1984; Schon, 1991), who suggest that practitioners have to deal with the totality of the problems as they are presented in practice and cannot readily find answers in the literature to these issues. Such problems cannot be solved by means of technical rational solutions.

Reed and Robbins (1991) suggest that nursing models were introduced as a starting point for the development of nursing theory. However, nursing models are grand theories, which encompass all aspects of nursing and thus seem to be inappropriate within practice. The adoption of nursing models has become widespread in nursing with little empirical evidence of their usefulness or critical evaluation. Roper et al. (1996) proposed a model of nursing which focuses on activities of living; it is derived from twelve components. They believe there is a lack of written evidence on the thinking and decision making of nurses and because of this nursing can often be undervalued and misunderstood.

Roper et al. (1996) suggested that nurses' commitment of their actions to paper would provide the evidence of a body of knowledge for nursing. This, in turn, would give value to the effectiveness of nursing care. The literature and nursing practice does not, however, suggest that this is the case. There does now seem to be a problem with nursing models and also problems attributed to a lack of understanding regarding the major issues of the models by nurses themselves. Some suggest this could be due to a lack of education in the initial introduction of nursing models to nurses (Reed, 1992).

As part of a larger study, Reed (1992) analysed the Kardex and care plans on three wards responsible for care of older people. Reed identified problems using nursing models that did not match the patients' problems. Therefore, the assumption that nursing is problem solving does not always match the aims of nursing, for example, in long-term older people's care. Models that seek to break down patients into sections are likely to result in problems of category fit. Reed's study suggested that there were practical problems of locating relevant data; and there were the much more crucial issues of what these data actually indicated about the way in which the nurses assessed their patients.

The care plans and written documentation did not reflect the complex and individual nursing care actually practised in older people's nursing which related to formal and final causes. Benner and Wrubel (1989) have suggested that the term 'model' is mechanistic and derived from the natural sciences. They suggest that when this is used on the non-human world and objects the result can be an increased understanding. However, if used in human inquiry the results can be confusing, and lacking in understanding. Nursing models seek to make nursing more manageable but in doing so fail to define what nursing is because they do not truly reflect the 'theories in action' of those nurses. Roper et al. (1996) hoped to achieve consensus as to the beliefs and goals and practice of nursing that are common. This drive towards uniformity may have inappropriately assumed that nursing remains the same in similar situations.

Nolan et al. (2004) discuss person-centred care as a new vision for gerontological nursing. The sense framework captures the individual and subjective nature and dimensions of caring relationships, and represents a middle-range nursing theory. The framework (Nolan, 2004) is underpinned by the belief that all staff involved in caring and the older person, carers and voluntary carers, should experience relationships that promote a sense of security, belonging, continuity, purpose, achievement and significance if high standards of nursing care are to be reached. The framework advocated by Nolan has been the subject of extensive empirical testing. Nolan suggests that therapeutic care requires a shared understanding and to do this we have to use the same language and concepts. This is very important in relation to vulnerable older people. Nolan discusses care of older people's needs to take account of the individual interpretations of experience. The framework presented in this book, the author believes, is broadly similar to the framework advocated by Nolan in that it totally considers the individual nature of each episode of care in a nursing situation.

Nursing care of the older person – a unique experience

Nursing practice in care of older people in this study demonstrated how each situation is uniquely different. It was not possible to have uniformity in the practice situation. Each nurse was dealing with an individual patient with his or her own personal needs. Nursing models do not deal with what nursing is, but with what nursing should be. There is a clear divide between the two. The nurses found the model of nursing (Roper et al., 1996) tended to complicate rather than assist nursing practice. An analysis of nursing theory has indicated that there are many problems associated with both deductive and speculative nursing theories, since both forms of theory are based on the premise that theory should be developed formal research and transmitted to nurses. There are tensions that exist within nursing around the appropriateness of nursing theory in its present form. The main issue that seemed to require addressing is the level of nursing theory that is actually the most compatible with the 'theory in action' used by nurses in the clinical situation.

The language of nursing theory, as written in the nursing literature, was different from what was used in practice. It was not only the language but also the words that were different. The differences in the speech and language prevented the nurses from using the literature. The practice that they know and talk about with their colleagues was not recognised as having the same meaning, or written with meaning about practice.

Theory building from the practice of older people's nursing

In this book the author has talked about how an alternative approach to theory development was used in the study which sought not to test hypotheses but to describe and explain the informal practice theories of nurses in older people's nursing. The informal practice theory identified in this research acknowledged the social world in which nursing care of the older person was taking place. Hence, the new knowledge generated should be more relevant than grand nursing theories, as the practice theory isolated has emerged from practice itself.

The significance of the informal practice theories is that the nurses are constantly solving problems for practice and in doing so are constructing informal theories which are being constantly tested, modified and re-tested, and therefore on-the-spot validation of their own theorising occurs. The notion of informal theory testing, which refers to personal, individual theories about specific individual theories, has been noted by others (Benner, 1984; Rolfe et al., 2001). Educationalists Carr and Kemmis (1986) pointed out that informal theory is contained in practice by definition because without it, practice is merely random and uncoordinated activity. Informal theory and practice are linked by the uniqueness of nursing care. Benner (1984) noted the expertise with which nurses handled situations and referred to the notion of reflection in action in the development of personal, individual theories about specific patient situations.

Benner did not fully explore the informal practice theories through reflection in action and the ways that nurses formulated and tested informal theories in practice. There are features noted here that are different from those of Benner's notion of expertise. Benner's research proposed that there were distinct stages of novice to expert practice in nursing and a nurse's level of theorising in action was based on the length of their experience. In Benner's study only expert nurses were proposed to be developing theory in action in this way. The process of reflection in action is seen by all the nurses in the author's study as central to learning situations in the care of older patients. This was linked to their actions and on-the-spot experimenting as an attribute to professional nursing practice. There was evidence that this was the case for all of the nurses despite differences in qualifications and levels of experience in care of older patients. The way that nurses are developing their informal theories in action and on action seemed to demonstrate the notion of the cycle of theorising in action and praxis.

Developing this point further, the author would suggest that the concept of the practitioner is very important in the development and wider discussion on nursing theory in care of older people. The technical rationality model is not suitable for practice-based knowledge because practice is individual and contextualised. Schon (1991) argued that this paradox can be resolved by acknowledging the importance of subjectivity – for example, by reflecting on our actions and by granting inductive research equal status with deductive research – and that nursing theory could and should be developed from the informal theory model, with each nurse being recognised as in his or her own practice. Using Schon's analogy, the practitioner who is constantly using reflection in action as a means of generating theory and for practice would or could be seen as the nurse practitioner.

The recognition of informal theory as inductive theory building does not compromise the position of formal propositional theory – in fact, quite the opposite – and it is suggested that it would strengthen the relationship between practice and theory and help to close any gap between theory and practice. Usher and Bryant (1997) suggest utilising action research to capture the practice component of informal practice theory, which integrates formal and informal theory, reflection in action, reflection on action.

Inductive research of the kind that considers the informal theory cycle in practice is superior to traditional inductivism and hypthetico-deductivism for theory building. The traditional scientific positivist research is inadequate for theory generation in a practice-based discipline of nursing. This is because each nursing situation is about individual people and practice. Inductive theory building from practice is context specific, relating to particular situations in practice. Formal theory is different because it relates to global situations and exists independently of practice.

The informal practice theory in this book relates to the social world in which older people's nursing care was taking place. The significance of the factors isolated and the relationships between them was that the nurses were constantly solving problems for practice and in doing so were constructing their own informal theories which were being constantly tested, modified and re-tested; therefore validation of their own theorising was occurring. Indeed, the notion of informal theory testing which refers to personal, individual theories about specific individual theories has been noted by others (Carr, 1986; Rolfe, 1999, 2001).

Conclusion

The importance of informal theory is that the practitioner is able to solve problems in practice, through a process of testing, modifying, re-testing and experimenting there and then in practice. This seems to be the difference between the relationship of formal theory and informal practice theory and has not been given enough recognition or development. The relationship between informal theory and practice is constant with practice generating theory, and theory modifying practice. In this way, each nurse was building up their own understanding in situations which were being modified in new nursing situations.

Suggested reading

Eraut, M. (1994) *Developing Professional Knowledge and Competence* (London: Falmer Press). The author offers an original analysis of professional knowledge and professional learning. The book brings together theory and practice, the balance between analysis and intuition in making decisions, and the roles of different types of knowledge.

Ham, C. (2004) *Health Policy in Britain the Politics and Organisation of the National Health Service*, 5th edition (Basingstoke: Palgrave Macmillan). This book examines and analyses the approaches taken by successive governments to the reform of the NHS. It is a leading text on British health policy.

Levin, P. (1997) *Making Social Policy: The Mechanisms of Government and Politics, and How to Investigate Them* (Buckingham: Open University Press). Starting from first principles, this book examines policy through concepts drawn directly from the experiences and perceptions of politicians. Includes case studies.

Schon, D. (1991) *The Reflective Practitioner* (New York: Basic Books). A classic text from the general education literature. It offers new insights into practice-based theories. Well worth reading.

Thompson, N. (1995) *Theory and Practice in Health and Social Welfare* London: Open University Press). This book is an important and timely exploration of many of the key issues around the integration of theory and practice. It presents a sensible approach to theory and practice, geared towards improving practice. The author argues the case for making theory relevant to practice.

Future trends: standards and quality in care

This chapter:

▶ considers the future care of older people;
▶ outlines global health issues for older people;
▶ discusses modern and contemporary changes in practice for older people.

Changing needs

Chapter 7 describes the changing needs of older people in society and will focus on how nurses will be able to meet the needs of older people in response to the policies on care of older people. This chapter will look at care of older people in the future, examining global health issues and the challenges to be met in terms of how there is a need to achieve world-class standards for older people in key services. The implications for research in the study of future practice of care of older people are discussed.

Empowerment for older people

There are challenges facing nurses in both primary and secondary care. Populations are aging in developed countries and there are increased demands for resources and services. Nurses working with older people are key players in encouraging healthy lifestyles, and integrated approaches are essential to good standards of nursing care. There is a great need to plan ahead for the ageing population in order to improve the quality of services offered to older people. In its document *A Sure Start to Later Life* (DoH, 2006a) the Department of Health looks at a new way of working for care of older people in the future, and suggests a new economics of empowerment for older people that would benefit the individual and society in general. This shows that there needs to be a shift to a participatory model, and from crisis management to prevention and wellbeing, which includes physical and social activities to protect health. We already know that inactivity and isolation of the individual seem to accelerate physical and social decline. Physical activity is important to improve strength, balance and co-ordination. *A Sure Start to Later Life* advocates a shift: to start with the individual and not the service in order to ensure empowerment of the older person. Older people consider improved wellbeing and quality of life as important issues.

Dignity in care

The Department of Health (2006b) launched a new campaign in care of older people relating to dignity of care. It suggests that health and social services have made good progress in driving down waiting lists and improving access to services. However, the emphasis on throughput might in some way have had a detrimental effect on the quality of care provided for older people and their families.

The Dignity in Care campaign has attempted to raise awareness of the need for dignity in care, and to spread best practice and support health and social care staff to improve standards for older people. These suggestions cover some of the key areas that are regarded as having importance:

- support people with the same respect you would want for yourself or a member of your family;
- treat each person as an individual;
- enable people to maintain the maximum possible degree of independence;
- listen and support people;
- respect people's right to privacy;
- ensure people feel able to complain;
- engage with family members and carers;
- help people to maintain confidence and a positive self-esteem;
- act to alleviate people's loneliness and isolation.

The above points are regarded by the Department of Health (2006b) as the basis of high-quality services that respect people's dignity. The challenge to ensure dignity in care could be seen as part of the much wider issue of the ways in which behaviour and standards in society are changing.

There seems to be a new strategic vision and direction for working with older people that can provide a greater sense of therapeutic care, which involves working in partnership with older people. The Royal College of Nursing (2006) identified a set of core principles which underpin good nursing practice. In essence these were:

- valuing older people;
- maximising potential by working with people to help to recognise their potential;
- ensuring good quality by meeting the needs of the whole person;
- enabling through information: sharing information with older people and their carers by working in partnership.

Pause for thought

How have the changes in policy, as discussed above, influenced your practice of caring for older people?

The National Office for Statistics has figures that show there is an increase in the percentage of older people within communities, which is set to increase (see Soule et al., 2005). Patterns of disease are changing, the burden shifting to the old with chronic conditions. This is reflected in increased admissions to hospital, increasing waiting times and delays with an over-reliance on the secondary care services. World-class healthcare is a global issue where healthcare is supported by a social care system. Services in the future will mean working in partnership with all stakeholders. Moving from a task-based systems approach to working and engaging with the individual and their family is a must. This provides opportunities for nurses to draw on the capacity of carers, families and voluntary and self-help groups in primary care. Nurses will be key players in the future to develop services and set up networks to make this happen.

Clearly, with the ageing population in developed countries set to rise, there is an ever-increasing demand for resources and services to meet the needs of older people in society. It is likely that in the future the demands on nurses will change because, as the population age and experience more long-term conditions, the care that nurses provide will necessarily become more complex.

The National Service Framework (NSF) for older people (DoH, 2001) has already had a major effect in setting up national standards of care for older people in the UK. There are two principles which are inherent in the NHS: the promotion of person-centred care, and the rooting out of age discrimination in the NHS. Nolan et al. (2004) recommended that nurses consider client centredness as the watchword for quality care in the twenty-first century. Patient-, client- or person-centred care reflects the emergence of new ways of working with older people both in primary and in secondary care in a range of environments. The focus on patients' individuality reflects wider and broader trends within health and social care, which Nolan emphasises, stressing the importance of promoting the independence and autonomy of older people by greater user involvement.

Nolan suggests a move to relationship-centred care. This is in keeping with McCormack and McCance (2006), who believe that the essence of nursing lies in the nature of the nurse–patient relationship. This means that nurses are more empowering for older people in this type of philosophy for care. Indeed, good quality and standard of nursing care is best understood in terms of the nurse–patient and family relationship and there is a need to understand the similarities of the features of these and those evident in the framework identified in this book. In this book, the author has shown that nurses are able to maximise their skills by working in a therapeutic way to engage with older people and to maximise their quality of life.

Nolan et al. (2004) suggest the sense framework. The older person, family carers and paid voluntary carers should experience a sense of:

- *security* – to feel safe within relationships;
- *belonging* – to feel part of things;
- *continuity* – to experience links and consistency;
- *purpose* – to have a personally valuable goal;
- *achievement* – to make progress towards a desired goal;
- *significance* – to feel that you matter.

Any framework for work with older people needs to ensure that people experience interactions.

Nursing in care of older people

The main issue in nursing is that nursing is concerned with viewing the patient as a whole, with an emphasis upon the individual's own perspective of their experience. Nursing by this account is about a nurturing response of one to another in need, and it involves a nurse–patient relationship. Being able to focus on significant events, conditions or situations is central to nursing practice. Having an unconditional positive regard for the other person, together with the integrity to focus on significant events and situations, allows each nurse to acknowledge the problems of the patient. Nurses develop an ability to understand the importance of certain events and put them into context, therefore developing a deep meaning of shared experience between them and their patient. It appears that nursing as caring has been developed in a holistic way so that older patients are recognised as people with physical, psychological and social needs.

Focusing on the nature of everyday nursing care of older people should allow us to understand the nature and meaning of nursing care from both the scientific, demonstrable perspective and the invisible, complex, intangible and cultural perspective. The research study that this book is based on has shown that nursing knowledge reveals nursing practice to be contextual and formed by specific situations in particular times and places.

The nature of nursing relates to complex issues which involve the enhancement of the wellbeing of the person being nursed. It also relates to the nurse–patient relationship as a central pivot. The concept of caring in relation to the nature of nursing has been advocated as a therapy in its own right. Nursing is viewed as caring, which covers a range of physical, cognitive, moral and emotional behaviours that demand the presence of a nurse to sense the patient's needs and to respond to the patient with respect. Benner (1984) reminds us that nursing practice is shifting away from the traditional, systematically verified knowledge of empiricism, which does not represent the nature of nursing practice, towards a more holistic paradigm in order to develop a theory of nursing from practice. Clearly the main issue is about patient care, and ensuring nurses are able to respond individually, competently, professionally and morally in each nursing situation.

The Department of Health, in a document titled *A Recipe for Care – Not a Single Ingredient* (2007), describes how services need to change to keep up with demand. As seen in Chapter 3 of this book, by 2025 the number of people in the UK aged 85 will have increased by two-thirds. As older people are the main users of health and social care services, this means there are huge issues to address.

The number of people over 50 is projected to rise significantly until 2030 (see Figure 7.1). Therefore primary prevention and health promotion is essential. There should be a strong infrastructure to promote healthy lifestyles across communities, as well as working with the 50-plus population to promote shared responsibility for maintaining heath and wellbeing and, where necessary, early diagnosis through screening. There will need to be evidence-based chronic condition management, with practitioners working alongside individuals and their families and carers to empower people to manage their condition. The Chronic Conditions Model builds on evidence and developments to date from across the United Kingdom and internationally, and draws from the *International Overview of the Evidence on Effective Service Models in Chronic Disease Management* (DoH, 2006). The review demonstrated that important elements in achieving improved outcomes for people with chronic conditions were broad, managed care programmes; targeting high-risk people; sharing skills and knowledge; patient and carer involvement in decision making; self-managed education; self-monitoring telemedicine and telecare.

United Kingdom

Thousands

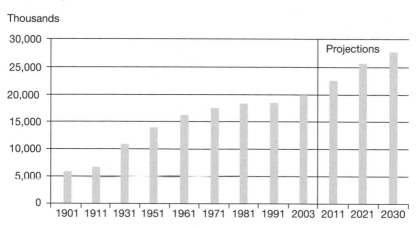

Figure 7.1 Number of people aged 50 and over (from the Office of Public Sector Information, reproduced with permission).

The Department of Health publication *Opportunity Age: Meeting the Challenges of Ageing in the 21st Century* (2005) discusses the main building blocks for quality of life as:

- standards of comparison and expectations;
- a positive attitude;
- good health;
- good social networks and sense of support;
- living in a neighbourhood with good facilities;
- feeling safe.

As the age profile of older people and the population changes, this evidence needs to be taken fully into account in developing future strategies.

Primary care and community nursing of older people

Primary care should provide key elements of older people's care, summarised as 'assessment of the person'. For management of long-term conditions in primary care, community nurses should find new ways of working to integrate with social care and specialist services. This should be in partnership with the older person and their carers. In essence, more personalised care and better co-ordination of services is important for future practice. Nursing older people will focus on evidence-based care and the effectiveness of interventions that support independence (Redfern, 2006).

The Future of Primary Care – Meeting the Challenges of the New NHS Market (Lewis and Dixon, 2005), which discusses the new contractual flexibilities and commissioning incentives in primary care, is likely to result in innovations in the provision and commissioning of services for older people. Many areas already offer services for chronic disease management and urgent out-of-hour care services. New roles in primary care will be developed with an overall aim to:

- improve the health of the community and to reduce health inequalities;
- secure the provision of safe, high-quality services;
- provide contract management of practices;
- engage with local people to hear patients' views and provide coherent access to health and social care.

Individual holistic assessment and person-centred care

The nursing care discussed in this book does match the policies being developed for care of older people as described above. In this instance there was a real opportunity to value individualised care and it means that nurses are in a good position to lead on policy issues and decisions about service provision for older people in their future practice.

Holistic assessment of older people involves working with the family and was seen as being significant. Older people were involved in their future care and this was considered an important issue in older people's nursing. Holistic assessment was seen to be in action and a constant part of nursing practice – not as a technical intervention or practical skill but also not as formal propositional protocols or standard plans. Any assessment tool that attempts to break down the human element into functional and mechanistic elements, as described in this book, is not going to address the empowering aspects of nursing care for older people, seen as desirable by policy makers.

Policy makers talk of capturing real experiences and of promoting a person-centred approach to current nursing. Practice that promotes a move forward towards person-centred care (McCormack and McCance, 2006) involves maximising the individual's potential within a nurse–patient relationship based on true companionship.

Developing an ethnography of older people

The discussion in this book has demonstrated the ways that nurses in the practice of older people's nursing have generated their own informal theories. The practice of older people's nursing has been made more visible for discussions about the practice of older people's nursing. It is possible that these theories are transferable to other nursing settings that nurses work in, in a more general way, and this indicates that there is an informal theory being generated in action by nurses.

This raises many possibilities for understanding and information about generating informal theories of nursing from nurses' practice. It opens the doors for nurses to look again at their practice, and to recognise that nurses can develop their own theories.

Pause for thought

Consider a nursing action that you have taken in patient care. How did you arrive at that decision or action? Where did you get the information or knowledge from? Why did you take that line of action? How would you perform in a similar situation in your future practice?

Finding one's way around qualitative methods in both the social sciences and nursing literature in itself sometimes presents unique challenges for nurses. The research presented in this book has brought into focus the differences in understanding between how the nurses were developing their informal theories and how the practitioners themselves generate theory in and on action. The work in this book has evolved from practice itself. It has very much related to individual patients and about individual problems in the context of care of older people, and was context specific. Therefore, informal practice theory is highly contextual and focused on individual practice as the nurse is encountering it. Informal theories developed from the practice situations, which were sometimes based on empirical or experiential knowledge, and sometimes a combination put together by the nurses themselves.

Ethnography of older people's nursing

In this research the ethnographic analysis went from a very broad remit in its early phase but became narrower and more focused as the research proceeded. In the first stage of the data analysis the author used a content analysis approach, which was guided by the qualitative literature. Finally, a set of factors emerged from the data analysis which came to play an important role in understanding the work of nurses working with older people.

Analysis moved from a structured and descriptive approach into a somewhat broader interpretation. The author gained understanding of the complex nature of practice theory and of the culture and meaning of the nurses' actions, and was guided by much of the literature on interpretive inquiry (Lincoln and Guba, 1985; Hammersley and Atkinson, 1995).

Typical and ordinary days in the care of older people

From this ethnography of older people's nursing the author has created an open and balanced interpretation of the nurses' practice. On reflection, the apparent lack of negative instances of practice has not been an oversight. The author did not, after all, set out to evaluate practice. The episodes of practice were described by some of the nurses as 'typical and ordinary days'. Although the author did not observe poor practice, there were, however, some situations where the nurses seemed to think they could have handled situations better, or at least they might have if they had had more resources. They were short of staff at times: this was a common problem on most wards and nursing practice areas, and nurses often talked about the lack of time and resources. The author's interpretation of situations often related to the tremendous number of details that the nurses were dealing with at one time in sometimes very difficult situations.

Box 7.1   Reflexive notes

Author's reflexivity: final thoughts

I believe I have, in common with many ethnographers, an etic and emic research style. I have shared the subjective meaning held by the nurses together with their culturally specific model. This has been developed using my own reflexive analysis of the data from the perspectives made explicit by the nurses. Adopting a critical reflexive perspective helped them to solve problems in practice.

At the start of this book the author reflected on her initial interest in studying practice theory in nursing that arose when, as a nurse educator, she was faced with unexplained incidents from students' stories of their practice. It was not possible to support nurses' accounts with theoretical explanations. The author therefore set out to explain and to explore theories of practice of older people's nursing.

The significance of recognising that reflection in action was occurring within the practice of care of older people was that there was a construction of informal theories, which were being tested, modified and re-tested with on-the-spot experimenting in action.

A significant area of information that emerged was that the factors identified in this account were not shown in the nursing literature. They were generated from nursing practice itself, and were contextualised to individual nursing situations. It does appear that nursing theorists have been developing grand nursing theories without addressing the 'on the spot' decision making that is happening in practice situations (Meyers, 2000; McCormack and McCance, 2006).

This book illustrates the value of nurse researchers recognising the actions of nurses and the ways in which informal practice theories are developed by reflection in and on action. The process of observing practice does present methodological issues for consideration but, like many experiences in research, it presents challenges for the development of quality nursing standards for the future. Nurses should have the opportunity in future research to develop informal practice theories through an in-depth evaluation of other specialties in nursing, and to explore informal practice in those areas of their own practice. Action research is particularly suited to identifying problems in clinical practice, and helping to solve issues in order to improve nursing practice (Meyers, 2000).

Practitioner-based research is well recognised in the field of general education. The superiority of professional judgement as opposed to the technical rationality model is well documented in teaching. In nursing there has been a tremendous effort to develop a formal theory of nursing as grand and middle-range theories without acknowledgement being made of practice theory in the way that informal practitioners themselves are generating theory (Meleis, 2006). This book has shown that there needs to be more recognition of practitioner-based research. Inductive research provides a framework to build a knowledge base for nursing because the informal theory is emerging from practice itself.

Conclusion

Nursing should be recognised as an inherent human process that is subjective and involving complexities. The way in which nurses engage with the older person and their family to assist with these complexities is the essence of nursing practice itself. The nature of nursing as a process of nourishing and promoting the development or progress of the patient represents the practice of nursing for each individual patient.

Suggested reading

Benner, P., Tanner, C. A. and Chesla, C. A. (1996) *Expertise in Nursing Practice: Caring, Clinical Judgement and Ethics* (New York: Springer Publishing Company). This volume analyses and examines the nature of clinical knowledge and judgement. A research study using clinical narratives to refine the stages of clinical skills acquisition and the components of expert practice.

Usher, R., Bryant, I. and Johnston, R. (1997) *Adult Education and the Post-modern Challenge: Learning beyond the Limits*. London: Routledge. This book examines how knowledge is viewed in society. The challenges of post-modernism and the creation of knowledge from practice are posed. Well worth reading.

Wanless, D. (2006) (London: King's Fund). This strategic report was awarded Prospect think tank 'Publication of the Year 2006'. It gets to the heart of the issues and opens up the debate about what social care will do in the future for older people.

References

Preface

Argyris, C. and Schon, D. (1974) *Theory into Practice: Increasing Professional Effectiveness*. San Francisco: Jossey Bass.

Carper, B. A. (1978) Fundamental patterns of knowing in nursing. *Advances in Nursing Science* 1 (1): 13–23.

Johns, C. (1996) Visualising and realising caring in practice through guided reflection. *Journal of Advanced Nursing* 24 (6): 1135–43.

Meizirow, J. (1990) *Fostering Critical Reflection in Adulthood*. San Francisco: Jossey Bass.

Rolfe, G., Freshwater, D. and Jasper, J. (2001) *Critical Reflection for Nursing and the Helping Professions: A User's Guide*. London: Palgrave Macmillan.

Schon, D. (1991) *The Reflective Practitioner*. New York: Basic Books.

Introduction

Department of Health (2004) *Better Health in Old Age: Report*. London: DoH.

1 An ethnography of older people's nursing

Benner, P. (1984) *From Novice to Expert: Excellence in Clinical Nursing Practice*. Menlo Park, CA: Addison-Wesley.

Carper, B. A. (1978) Fundamental patterns of knowing in nursing. *Advances in Nursing Science* 1 (1): 13–23.

Denzin, N. and Lincoln, Y. S. (2005) *Handbook of Qualitative Research*, 3rd edition. Thousand Oaks, CA: Sage.

Dickoff, J. and James, P. (1968a) A theory of theories: a position paper. *Nursing Research* 17 (3): 197–203.

Dickoff, J. and James, P. (1968b) Researching researcher's role in theory development. *Nursing Research* 17 (4): 197–203.

Dickoff, J., James, P. and Wiedenbach, E. (1968) Theory in a practice discipline: Part I Practice orientated theories. *Nursing Research* 17 (5): 415–35.

Ebbutt, D. (1985) Educational action research: some general concerns and specific quibbles. In R. G. Burgess (ed.), *Issues in Educational Research: Qualitative Methods*. Lewes: Falmer Press.

Elliott, J. (1991) *Action Research for Educational Change*. Milton Keynes: Open University Press.

Eraut, M. (1994) *Developing Professional Knowledge and Competence*. London: Falmer Press.

Finlay, L. and Gough, B. (2003) *Reflexivity: A Practical Guide For Researchers in Health and Social Sciences*. Oxford: Blackwell Publishing.

Hammersley, M. and Atkinson, P. (1995) *Ethnography: Principles in Practice*, 2nd edition. London: Routledge.

Jacox, A. K. (1974) Theory construction in nursing: an overview. *Nursing Research* 23 (1): 4–13.

Jamieson, A. and Victor, C. (2002) *Researching Ageing and Later Life*. London: Open University Press.

Johns, C. (1996) Visualising and realising caring in practice through guided reflection. *Journal of Advanced Nursing* 24 (6): 1135–43.

Lawler, J. (1991) *Behind the Screens: Nursing, Somology and the Problems of the Body*. London: Churchill Livingstone.

Lincoln, Y. S. and Guba, E. G. (1985) *Naturalistic Enquiry*. Newbury Park, CA: Sage Publications.

Meerabeau, E. (1992) Tacit nursing knowledge: an untapped resource or a methodological headache? *Journal of Advanced Nursing* 17 (1): 108–12.

Meleis, A. I. (1995) Role insufficiency and role supplementation: a conceptual framework. *Nursing Research* 24 (4): 254–71.

Meleis, A. I. (2006) *Theoretical Nursing: Development and Progress*, 4th edition. London: Lippincott Williams and Wilkins.

Polit, D. and Beck, C. (2004) *Nursing Research Principles and Methods*, 7th edition. London: Lippincott Williams and Wilkins.

Schon, D. (1991) *The Reflective Practitioner*. New York: Basic Books.

Silverman, D. (2006) *Interpreting Qualitative Data: Methods for Analysing Talk, Text and Interaction*, 3rd edition. London: Sage.

2   Theory development in nursing

Argyris, C. and Schon, D. (1974) *Theory into Practice: Increasing Professional Effectiveness*. San Francisco: Jossey Bass.

Benner, P. (1984) *From Novice to Expert: Excellence in Clinical Nursing Practice*. Menlo Park, CA: Addison-Wesley.

Benner, P. (1994) *Interpretive Phenomenology: Embodiment, Caring, and Ethics in Health and Illness*. London: Sage Publications.

Benner, P. and Wrubel, J. (1989) *The Primacy of Caring: Stress and Coping in Health and Illness*. Menlo Park, CA: Addison-Wesley.

Carper, B. A. (1978) Fundamental patterns of knowing in nursing. *Advances in Nursing Science* 1 (1): 13–23.

Carr, W. (1986) Theories of theory and practice. *Journal of Philosophy of Education* 20 (2): 177–86.

Carr, W. and Kemmis, S. (2002) *Becoming Critical: Education Knowledge and Action Research*. London: Falmer Press.

Davies, S. (2005) Meleis's theory of nursing transitions and relatives' experiences of nursing home entry. *Journal of Advanced Nursing* 52 (6): 658–71.

Davies, S. and Nolan, M. B. (2006) Making it better: self-perceived roles of family care givers of older people living in care homes; a qualitative study. *International Journal of Nursing Studies* 43 (2): 281–91.

Department of Health (2005) *Research Governance Framework for Health and Social Care*, 2nd edition. London: Department of Health.

Dickoff, J. and James, P. (1968) A theory of theories: a position paper. *Nursing Research* 17 (3): 197–203.

Elliott, J. (1991) *Action Research for Educational Change*. Milton Keynes: Open University Press.

Eraut, M. (1994) *Developing Professional Knowledge and Competence*. London: Falmer Press.

Fawcett, J. (1984) *Metaparadigm Analysis and Evaluation of Conceptual Models of Nursing*. Philadelphia, PA: F. A. Davis.

Hammersley, M. and Atkinson, P. (1995) *Ethnography: Principles in Practice*, 2nd edition. London: Routledge.

Jacox, A. K. (1974) Theory construction in nursing: an overview. *Nursing Research* 23 (1): 4–13.

Johns, C. (1996) Visualising and realising caring in practice through guided reflection. *Journal of Advanced Nursing* 24 (6): 1135–43.

Johnson, D. E. (1980) The behavioural systems model for nursing. In J. P. Rhyl and C. Roy (eds), *Conceptual Models for Nursing Practice*. London. Appleton-Century-Crofts.

King, I. (1981) *A Theory for Nursing: Systems, Concepts, Process*. New York: Wiley.

Kolb, D. A. (1985) *Learning Style Inventory: Technical Manual*. Boston, MA: McBer.

Leininger, M. M. (1991) Transcultural care principles, human rights and ethical considerations. *Journal of Transcultural Nursing* 3 (1): 25–30.

Lewin, K. (1958) *Readings in Social Psychology*. London: Holt Rinehart and Winston.

Lincoln, Y. S. and Guba, E. G. (1985) *Naturalistic Enquiry*. Newbury Park, CA: Sage Publications.

McCormack, B. and McCance, T. (2006) Development of a framework for person-centred nursing. *Journal of Advanced Nursing* 56 (5): 472–9.

McKay, A. (1969) Theories, models and systems for nursing. *Nursing Research* 18 (5): 393–9.

Meerabeau, E. (1992) Tacit nursing knowledge: an untapped resource or a methodological headache? *Journal of Advanced Nursing* 17 (1): 108–12.

Meizirow, J. (1990) *Fostering Critical Reflection in Adulthood*. San Francisco: Jossey Bass.

Meleis, A. I. (1997) *Theoretical Nursing: Development and Progress*, 3rd edition. Philadelphia, PA: Lippincott.

Meleis, A. I. (2006) *Theoretical Nursing: Development and Progress*, 4th edition. London: Lippincott Williams and Wilkins.

Menzies, I. (1960) A case study in the functioning of social systems as a defence against anxiety. *Human Relationships* 13 (1): 95–121.

Morse, J. M. (1995) Exploring the theoretical basis of nursing using advanced techniques of concept analysis. *Advances in Nursing Science* 17 (3): 31–46.

Nightingale, F. (1986) *Notes on Nursing – What It Is and What It Is Not*. New York: Dover Publications.

Orem, D. E. (2001) *Nursing: Concepts of Practice*, 5th edition. St Louis: Mosby.

Peplau, H. E. (1988) *Interpersonal Relations in Nursing*. New York: Putman.

Polanyi, M. (1967) *The Tacit Dimension*. London: Routledge and Kegan Paul.

Polit, D. F., Beck, C. T. and Hungler, B. P. (2001) *Essentials of Nursing Research. Methods, Appraisal, and Utilization*, 5th edition. Philadelphia, PA: Lippincott.

Reed, J. and Robbins, I. (1991) Models of nursing: their relevance to the care of elderly people. *Journal of Advanced Nursing* 16 (11): 1350–57.

Rogers, M. E. (1970) *An Introduction to the Theoretical Basis of Nursing*. Philadelphia: F. A. Davis.

Rolfe, G. (1999) Insufficient evidence: the problems of evidence-based nursing. *Nurse Education Today* 19 (6): 433–42.

Rolfe, G., Freshwater, D. and Jasper, M. (2001) *Critical Reflection for Nursing and the Helping Professions: A User's Guide*. Hampshire: Palgrave.

Roy, C. (1984) *Introduction to Nursing: An Adaptation Model*, 2nd edition . Englewood Cliffs, NJ: Churchill Livingstone.

Royal College of Nursing (1996a) *The Royal College of Nursing Clinical Effectiveness Initiative: A Strategic Framework*. London: RCN.

Royal College of Nursing (1996c) *Clinical Effectiveness: A Royal College of Nursing Guide*. London: RCN.

Royal College of Nursing (2005) *Research Governance Framework for Health and Social Care*, 2nd edition. London: RCN.

Ryle, G. (1949) *The Concept of Mind*. Chicago: University of Chicago Press.

Schon, D. (1990) *Educating the Reflective Practitioner*. San Francisco: Jossey Bass.

Schon, D. (1991) *The Reflective Practitioner*. New York: Basic Books.

Silverman, D. (2006) *Interpreting Qualitative Data: Methods for Analysing Talk, Text and Interaction*, 3rd edition. London: Sage.

Stenhouse, L. (1975) *An Introduction to Curriculum Research and Development*. Oxford: Heinemann.

Usher, R., Bryant, I. and Johnston, R. (1997) *Adult Education and the Post Modern Challenge: Learning Beyond the Limits*. London: Routledge.

Walker, L. and Avant, V. (1994) *Strategies for Theory Construction in Nursing,* 3rd edition. Norwalk, CT: Appleton and Lange.

Walsh, M. and Ford, P. (1990) *Nursing Rituals.* Oxford: Butterworth-Heinemann.

Watson, J. (1988) *Nursing: Human Science and Human Care.* Norwalk, Ct: Appleton-Century-Crofts; New York: National League for Nursing.

Webster, G., Jacox, A. and Baldwin, B. (1981) Nursing theory and the ghost of the received view. In J. C. McCloskey and H. K. Grace (eds), *Current Issues in Nursing.* Boston, MA: Blackwell Scientific Publications.

Wolf, Z. R. (1993) The bath: a nursing ritual. *Journal of Holistic Nursing* 11 (2): 135–48.

3   Building professional knowledge in older people's care

Baker, D. (1978) Attitudes of nurses to the care of the elderly. PhD dissertation, University of Manchester.

Beveridge, W. H. (1942) *Social Insurance and Allied Services.* London: Inter-Departmental Committee.

Charmaz, K. (2006) *Constructing Grounded Theory: A Practical Guide Through Qualitative Analysis.* London: Sage Publications.

Davies, S. and Nolan, M. B. (2006) Making it better: self-perceived roles of family care givers of older people living in care homes; a qualitative study. *International Journal of Nursing Studies* 43 (2): 281–91.

Dellasega, C. and Curriero, F. (1991) The effects of institutional and community experiences on nursing students' intentions towards work with the elderly. *Journal of Nurse Education* 30 (9): 405–10.

Department of Health (2001) *National Service Framework for Older People.* London: Department of Health.

Department of Health (2004) *The NHS Improvement Plan: Putting People at the Heart of Public Services.* Norwich: Department of Health.

Department of Health (2006) *'Dignity in Care' Public Survey: Report on People's Views.* London: Department of Health.

Evers, H. (1981) Tender loving care? – Patients and nurses in geriatric wards. In L. A. Copp (ed.), *Nursing Elderly People.* London: Churchill Livingstone.

Fagerberg, I. (1998) Nursing students' narrated lived experiences of caring, education and the transition into nursing focusing on care of the elderly. PhD dissertation , Stockholm University.

Goffman, E. (1961) *Asylums.* New York: Doubleday Anchor.

Herdman, E. (2002) Challenging the discourses of nursing ageism. *International Journal of Nursing Studies* 39: 1105–14.

McCormack, B. (2004) Person centredness in gerontological nursing: an overview of the literature. *International Journal of Older People Nursing* 13 (3a): 31–8.

McCormack, B. and McCance, T. (2006) Development of a framework for person-centred nursing. *Journal of Advanced Nursing* 56 (5): 472–9.

Melanson, P. M. and Downe-Wamboldt, B. L. (1985) Antecedents of Baccalaureate student nurses' attitudes towards the elderly. *Journal of Advanced Nursing* 10 (6): 527–32.

Morse, J. M. (1995) Exploring the theoretical basis of nursing using advanced techniques of concept analysis. *Advances in Nursing Science* 17 (3): 31–46.

Murray, K. (2002) Poor quality of elderly care deterring students *Nursing Standard* 29: 7.

Nolan, M. R., Keady, J. and Grant, G. (1995) Developing a typology of family care: implications for nurses and other service providers. *Journal of Advanced Nursing* 21 (2): 256–65.

Nolan, M. R., Davies, S., Brown, J., Keady, J. and Nolan, J. (2004) Beyond person centred care: a new vision for gerontological nursing. *International Journal of Older People Nursing* 13 (2a): 45–53.

Norton, D. (1975) *An Investigation of Geriatric Nursing Problems in Hospitals.* Edinburgh: Churchill Livingstone.

Portner, M. (2008) *Being Old Is Different: Person Centred Care for Older People.* Ross-on-Wye: PCCS Books.

Pursey, A. and Luker, K. (1995) Attitudes and stereotypes: nurses' work with older people. *Journal of Advanced Nursing* 22 (3): 547–55.

Royal College of Nursing (2004) *Caring in Partnership: Older People and Nursing Staff Working Towards the Future.* London: RCN.

Royal College of Nursing (2006) *Two Years On – Caring in Partnership: Older People and Nursing Staff Working Towards the Future.* London: RCN.

Savage, J. (1995) *Nursing Intimacy: An Ethnographic Approach to Nurse–Patient Interaction.* London: Scutari Press.

Slevin, O. (1991) Ageist attitudes among young adults: implications for a caring profession. *Journal of Advanced Nursing* 16 (11): 97–1205.

Smith, P. (1992) *The Emotional Labour of Nursing: How Nurses Care.* Basingstoke: Macmillan.

Stevens, J. A. and Crouch, M. (1992) Working with the elderly: do student nurses care for it? *Australian Journal of Advanced Nursing* 2 (3): 12–17.

Tudor-Hart, J. (1988) *A New Kind of Doctor.* London: Merlin Press.

Wells, T. J. (1980) *Problems in Geriatric Nursing Care.* Edinburgh: Churchill Livingstone.

4   The context and culture of the care setting

Audit Commission (2004) *Supporting Frail Older People: Independence and Wellbeing 3.* London: Audit Commission.

Department of Health (1997) *The New NHS, Modern, Dependable.* London: Stationery Office.

Department of Health (2001) *National Service Framework for Older People.* London: DoH.

Department of Health (2004) *Better Health in Old Age: Report.* London: DoH.

Department of Health (2006) *A New Ambition for Old Age: Next Steps in Implementing the National Service Framework for Older People.* London: DoH.

Department of Health (2007) *A Recipe for Care – Not a Single Ingredient.* London: DoH.

Elliott, J. (1991) *Action Research for Educational Change.* Milton Keynes: Open University Press.

Froggatt, K., Davis, S. and Meyer, J. (2009) *Understanding Care Homes – A Research and Development Perspective.* London: Jessica Kingsley.

King's Fund (2004) *Case-managing Long-term Conditions: What Impact Does It Have in the Treatment of Older People?* London: King's Fund.

King's Fund (2005) *Care Service Inquiry: Looking Forward to Care in Old Age – Expectations of the Next Generation.* London: King's Fund.

Nolan, M. R., Davies, S., Brown, J., Keady, J. and Nolan, J. (2004) Beyond person-centred care: a new vision for gerontological nursing. *International Journal of older People Nursing* 13 (2a): 45–53.

Reed (2006) Transition to a care home, the importance of choice and control. *Quality in Aging* 7 (4): 12–16.

Scottish Executive (2006) *Delivering Care, Enabling Health.* Edinburgh: Scottish Executive.

Smith, C. (2006) Who's looking after our old: who cares? *Nursing in Practice* July/August 2006 29: 22–4.

5   A framework for the delivery of care

Argyris, C. and Schon, D. (1974) *Theory into Practice: Increasing Professional Effectiveness.* San Francisco, CA: Jossey Bass.

Benner, P. (1984) *From Novice to Expert: Excellence in Clinical Nursing Practice.* Menlo Park, CA: Addison-Wesley.

Benner, P. and Wrubel, J. (1989) *The Primacy of Caring: Stress and Coping in Health and Illness.* Menlo Park, CA: Addison-Wesley.

Boud, D., Keogh, R. and Walker, D. (1985) *Reflection Turning Experience into Learning.* London: Kogan Page.

Campbell, A. (1984) *Moderated Love: A Theology of Professional Care.* London: S.P.C.K.

Carroll, (1993) *Caring for Older People – A Nurse's Guide.* London: Springer.

Department of Health (2006) *'Dignity in Care' Public Survey: Report on People's Views.* London: DoH.

Elliott, J. (1991) *Action Research for Educational Change.* Milton Keynes: Open University Press.

Ersser, S. and Tutton, E. (1991) *Primary Nursing in Perspective.* London: Scutari Press.

Gibb, H. and O'Brian, B. (1991) Jokes and reassurance are not enough: ways in which nurses relate through conversation with elderly clients. *Journal of Advanced Nursing* 15 (12): 1389–401.

Iliffe, S. and Drennan, V. (2003) Older people's services – a picture of health. *Health Service Journal* 113 (5852): 22–4.

Lawler, J. (1991) *Behind the Screens: Nursing, Somology and the Problems of the Body.* London: Churchill Livingstone.

McCormack, B. (2001) *Negotiating Partnerships with Older People: A Person Centred Approach.* Aldershot: Ashgate.

Meyers, J. (2000) Using qualitative methods in health related action research. *British Medical Journal* 15 320 (7228): 178–81.

Morse, J. M. (1983) An ethnographic analysis of comfort: a preliminary investigation. *Nursing Papers* 15 (1): 6–19.

Morse, J. M., Bottoroff, J. and Hutchinson, S. (1994) The phenomenology of comfort. *Journal of Advanced Nursing* 20 (1): 189–95.

Nolan, M. R., Davies, S., Brown, J., Keady, J. and Nolan, J. (2004) Beyond person-centred care: a new vision for gerontological nursing. *International Journal of older People Nursing* 13 (2a): 45–53.

Polanyi, M. (1956) *Personal Knowledge.* Chicago, IL: University of Chicago Press.

Redfern, S. and Ross, F. (2006) *Nursing Older People.* London: Churchill Livingstone.

Reed, J. and Robbins, I. (1991) Models of nursing: their relevance to the care of elderly people. *Journal of Advanced Nursing* 16 (11): 1350–57.

Rolfe, G., Freshwater, D. and Jasper, M. (2001) *Critical Reflection for Nursing and the Helping Professions: A User's Guide.* Hampshire: Palgrave.

Roper, N., Logan, W. and Tierney, A. (1983) *Using a Model for Nursing.* Edinburgh: Churchill Livingstone.

Royal Marsden Hospital (2004) *Clinical Nursing Procedures,* 6th edition. London: Blackwell Publications.

Schon, D. (1990) *Educating the Reflective Practitioner.* San Francisco, CA: Jossey Bass.

Schon, D. (1991) *The Reflective Practitioner.* New York: Basic Books.

Smith, P. (1992) *The Emotional Labour of Nursing: How Nurses Care.* Basingstoke: Palgrave Macmillan.

Smith, C. (2003) Researching the informal theories of nurses working with older people using a holistic, bio-psychosocial approach. *Quality in Ageing: Policy, Practice and Research* 4 (2): 36–47.

Smith, C., Snelgrove, S., Armstrong, Esther C. and Clark, J. (2003) Is there a future for the informal homecare of older people in a changing society? *Quality in Ageing: Policy Practice and Research* 4 (1): 82–91.

6   Focusing on the practice of caring for older people

Benner, P. (1984) *From Novice to Expert: Excellence in Clinical Nursing Practice.* Menlo Park, CA: Addison-Wesley.

Benner, P. and Wrubel, J. (1989) *The Primacy of Caring: Stress and Coping in Health and Illness*. Menlo Park, CA: Addison-Wesley.

Carr, W. (1986) Theories of theory and practice. *Journal of Philosophy of Education* 20 (2): 177–86.

Carr, W. and Kemmis, S. (1986) *Becoming Critical*. London: Routledge and Falmer Press.

Croche, B. (1920) *The Aesthetics and the Science of Expression and the Linguistics in General* (trans. 1992). Cambridge: Cambridge University Press.

Denzin, N. and Lincoln, Y. S. (2005) *Handbook of Qualitative Research*, 3rd edition. Thousand Oaks, CA: Sage.

Eraut, M. (1994) *Developing Professional Knowledge and Competence*. London: Falmer Press.

Lincoln, Y. S. and Guba, E. G. (1985) *Naturalistic Enquiry*. Thousand Oaks, CA: Sage Publications.

McCormack, B. (2003) A conceptual framework for person-centred practice with older people. *International Journal of Nursing Practice* 9 (3), 202–9.

McCormack, B. (2004) Person-centeredness in gerontological nursing: an overview of the literature. *Journal of Clinical Nursing* 13 (3a): 31–8.

Nolan, M. R., Davies, S., Brown, J., Keady, J. and Nolan, J. (2004) Beyond person-centred care: a new vision for gerontological nursing. *International Journal of older People Nursing* 13 (2a): 45–53.

Polanyi, M. (1967) *The Tacit Dimension*. London: Routledge and Kegan Paul.

Redfern, S. and Ross, F. (2006) *Nursing Older People*. London: Churchill Livingstone.

Reed, J. (1992) Secondary data in nursing research. *Journal of Advanced Nursing* 17 (1): 877–83.

Rolfe, G. (1999) Insufficient evidence: the problems of evidence-based nursing. *Nurse Education Today* 19 (8): 433–42.

Rolfe, G., Freshwater, D. and Jasper, J. (2001) *Critical Reflection for Nursing and the Helping Professions: A User's Guide*. London: Palgrave Macmillan.

Roper, N., Logan, W. W. and Tierney, A. J. (1996) *The Elements of Nursing: A Model for Nursing Based on a Model for Living*, 4th edition. Edinburgh: Churchill Livingstone.

Schon, D. (1990) *Educating the Reflective Practitioner*. San Francisco, CA: Jossey Bass.

Schon, D. (1991) *The Reflective Practitioner*. New York: Basic Books.

Taylor, C. (1985) *Philosophical Papers. Volumes 1 and 2*. In P. Benner and J. Wrubel (1989) *The Primacy of Caring: Stress and Coping in Health and Illness*. Menlo Park, CA: Addison-Wesley.

Usher, R., Bryant, I. and Johnston, R. (1997) *Adult Education and the Post-Modern Challenge: Learning Beyond the Limits*. London: Routledge.

Wittgenstein, L. (1967) *Philosophical Investigations*, 4th edition. Oxford: Blackwell.

7 Future trends: standards and quality in care

Benner, P. (1984) *From Novice to Expert: Excellence in Clinical Nursing Practice.* Menlo Park, CA: Addison-Wesley.

Department of Health (2001) *National Service Framework for Older People.* London: DoH.

Department of Health (2005) *Opportunity Age: Meeting the Challenges of Ageing in the 21st Century.* At: www.dwp.gov.uk

Department of Health (2006a) *A Sure Start to Later Life: Ending Inequalities for Older People: A Social Exclusion Final Report Department for Work and Pensions.* London: DoH.

Department of Health (2006b) *Dignity in Care: A Report on People's Views, What You Had to Say.* London: DoH.

Department of Health (2007) *A Recipe for Care – Not a Single Ingredient: Clinical Cases for Change: Report by Professor Ian Philp, National Director for Older People. NHS.* London: DoH.

Hammersley, M. and Atkinson, P. (1995) *Ethnography: Principles in Practice,* 2nd edition. London: Routledge.

Lewis, R. and Dixon, J. (2005) *The Future of Primary Care – Meeting the Challenges of the New NHS Market.* London: King's Fund.

Lincoln, Y. S. and Guba, E. G. (1985) *Naturalistic Enquiry.* Thousand Oaks, CA: Sage Publications.

McCormack, B. and McCance, T. (2006) Development of a framework for person-centred nursing. *Journal of Advanced Nursing* 56 (5): 472–9.

Meleis, A. I. (2006) *Theoretical Nursing: Development and Progress,* 4th edition. London: Lippincott Williams and Wilkins.

Meyers, J. (2000) Using qualitative methods in health-related action research. *British Medical Journal* 15 320 (7228): 178–81.

Nolan, R., Davies, S., Brown, J., Keady, J. and Nolan, J. (2004) Beyond person-centred care: a new vision for gerontological nursing. *International Journal of Older People Nursing* 13 (3a): 45–53.

Redfern, S. and Ross, M. (2006) *Nursing Older People,* 4th edition. London: Churchill Livingstone.

Royal College of Nursing (2006) *Caring in Partnership: Older People and Nursing Staff Working Towards the Future.* London: Royal College of Nursing.

Soule, A., Babb, P., Evandrou, M., Balchin, S. and Zealey, L. (2005) *National Statistics Focus on Older People.* http://www.statistics.gov.uk/focuson/olderpeople/

Index

Page numbers in *italics* refer to diagrams/tables

accountability issue 104–6
action research 39–40, 93, 124, 136
action theories 42, 87
activities of daily living (ADL) 73–4
acute secondary hospital care 66–8
Advanced Journal of Nursing 20
advising
  and nurse–patient relationship
    89–90
aesthetic knowledge 37
age discrimination 53, 129
ageing
  as factor in assessment process
    101–2
ageing population 65, 126, 128, 131,
  131
ageism 56, 60
analytic induction 17–19
annual health check 59
Argyris, C. 26, 42, 43, 98
art of nursing 36, 93, 99
assessment of patients 57, 59, 78, 90,
  91, 94, 97, 101–2, 118
association 99
Atkinson, P. 10, 11, 15, 17, 23, 38
Audit Commission Report (2004) 66
authority issue 104–6
autonomy issue 104–6

Baker, D. 55
bathing of patients 48–9
Benner, P. 27, 33–4, 35, 36, 83, 87, 95,
  96, 97, 99, 116, 121, 123, 130

Better Health in Old Age 3, 67
Beveridge Report (1942) 54
Boud, D. 43, 99
British Nursing Index (BNI) 20

Campbell, A. 83
care/caring 102–3
  dignity in 58, 59, 72, 96, 113,
    127–9
  distinction between caring about
    and caring for 101–2
  nursing as 102, 130
  philosophy of 77
care delivery framework 79–109, *80*
  accountability and autonomy in
    caring 104–6
  assessment of the home and
    family care 106–9
  caring and supporting 102–3
  collegial interactions 101
  love and companionship 103–4
  nurse–patient relationship 82–94
  nursing assessment 101–2
  nursing therapeutics 94–101
care plans 91–2, 96, 118–19, 121
carers 59, 72–4, 77, 100, 107
'carers as experts' model 77
Carers National Association 73
Carper, B. A. 37
Carr, W. 38–9, 40–1, 116, 123
case management 60, 71
Charmaz, K. 61
Chronic Conditions Model 131

chronic conditions/diseases 58, 66, 70, 128, 131
  and hospital admissions 67, 68
  number of people with 69
chronic disease management 131, 132
clinical effectiveness 46, 47, 49, 50
clinical reasoning 106
collegial interactions 101
comforting
  and nurse–patient relationship 92–3
commitment, nurses' 116
common meanings 35
communication skills 103–4
community care 59
community nurses/nursing 60, 68, 70, 72, 132
companionship 83, 102, 104, 133
concern
  and caring 102
content analysis 17, 18, 134
continuity of care 113–14
conversation styles 86–7
cost effectiveness
  stress on by NHS 47
critical incident analysis 26
critical thinking process 82, 90, 92, 106, 107
cross-infection 100
Cumulative Index for Nursing and Allied Health Literature (CINAHL) 20

Davies, S. 33, 34
Delivering Care, Enabling Health 70
Denzin, N. 11, 22, 111
Department of Health 20, 53, 60, 67, 72, 126, 127, 130, 132
descriptive theories 21, 45
Dickoff, J. 20, 21, 28, 31, 44–5
dignity in care 58, 59, 72, 96, 113, 127–9
'Dignity in Care' survey 58

district nurses 59, 71
documentation, nursing 91–2, 118–19, 121 see also care plans

education
  nurse 112, 114
  practice and theory in 29
elective healthcare 72
elimination care 96–7
Elliott, J. 39, 41–2, 76, 82
embodied knowledge 83
empathy 102
empirical knowledge 37
empiricism 130
empowerment, of older people 126–7
encouragement, of older patients 60, 86–8, 89, 96–7, 100, 113
Eraut, M. 113
espoused theory 42
ethics
  and knowing 37
  and researching care of older people 10–11
ethnography, of older people's nursing 9–10, 133–4
Evercare programme 60
evidence-based care 132
evidence-based knowledge 49–50
evidence-based practice 111
experiential learning 43, 114
expertise, nursing
  areas of practical knowledge observed in 35–6
explaining of care to older person 82–5

factor isolation 20–3, 22, 45
Fagerberg, I. 56
families
  involvement in patient care 107–8
  relationship between nurse and patients' 76–7, 90, 103, 107

family care situation, assessment of 104–6
family of practice 114, 116
fieldwork 10
Ford, P. 49
Future of Primary Care, The 132
future trends 126–36

General Medical Contract 59
generational gaps 70
geriatrics 54
Gibb, H. 86–7
Goffman, E. 54
grand nursing theories 27–8, 32, 40, 117, 120, 123, 136
grounded theory 61
Guba, E. G. 11, 111

Hammersley, M. 10, 11, 15, 17, 23, 38
health promotion 72
health and social policy 58–9
holistic approach 32, 103, 130, 133
home care 89, 105
home situation, assessment of 104–6
hospital care 74–7
    acute secondary 66–8
    admissions 60, 66, 75
    discharging patients from hospital 108
    involvement with patient families 76–7
    multidisciplinary team 75
    nurse–patient relationship 75–6, 77
    social dilemmas 76
    see also wards, hospital
hygiene care 94–6

incontinence 96
individual personal theories 115–16
inductive approach 34, 61, 111, 124, 136

informal practice theory 9–10, 23, 38–9, 40, 42–3, 115–16, 117, *117*, 122–3, 124, 134, 136
informal theory 2, 40, 46, 123, 124, 125, 133–4, 135
institutionalised care 54
integrated services 57–8
International Overview of the Evidence on Effective Service Models in Chronic Disease Management 131
interpretative approach 38, 134
interviews of nurses 12, 14–15
inverse care law 56

Jacox, A. K. 45
James, P. 20, 21, *28*, 31, 44–5
Johns, C. 18
Johnson, D. E. 32
journals, nursing 19–20, 114
judgements in action 90–2, 97

Kemmis, S. 38–9, 123
King, I. 32
King's Fund study 73
'know how' knowledge 36, 83, 95, 99, 116
'know that' knowledge 36
knowledge
    'know how' 36, 83, 95, 99, 116
    nursing 34–5
    and power 104
    practical 35–6, 39, 95, 97
    professional 34
    sources of in care of older people 114
    sources of in nursing 47–9
    tacit 44, 89, 95

labelling 21
Lawler, J. 85
Leininger, M. M. 32
Lincoln, Y. S. 11, 111
literature, nursing 19–20 *see also* journals, nursing

long-term conditions 70, 75
Luker, K. 56

McCance, T. 52, 53, 109, 117, 129
McCormack, B. 53, 89, 109, 117, 129
McKay, A. 28
maintenance
and older people's nursing 88–9
maxims 35
medical model of care 47–8
medications 98–9, 102
MEDLINE 20
Meerabeau, E. 44
Meizirow, J. 43
Meleis, A.I. 21, 28, 33
mentor system 114
Menzies, I. 37
Meyers, J. 93
middle-range nursing theory 33, 109, 121, 136
mobility/mobilisation 59, 86, 88, 89, 97, 100, 101
Morse, J. M. 34, 61, 93
multi-level systems model 32
multidisciplinary assessment 105
multidisciplinary team 75, 94

named nursing 75, 76, 104, 105–6, 108
naming theory 45
National Health Service see NHS
National Office for Statistics 128
National Service Framework (NSF) 58, 72, 129
National Service Framework for Older People 52–3, 58, 66
National Service Guidelines 3
New Ambition for Old Age, A 72
New NHS, The 67
NHS (National Health Service) 47, 129
Improvement Plan 60
Nightingale, F. 48
Nolan, M. R. 53, 57, 77, 121–2, 129

Norton, D. 54–5
nurse education 112, 114
nurse-managed beds 75
nurse–patient relationship 75–6, 79, 82–94, 103–4, 129, 130, 133
and advising 89–90
collaborating with multidisciplinary and interagency staff 94
and companionship 83, 102, 104, 133
encouragement of the older person 60, 86–8, 89, 96–7, 100, 113
ensuring comfort 92–3
explaining care to the older person 82–5
judgement in action at bedside 90–2
as key to successful nursing care 117
maintaining ability 88–9
working with patients' families 90
nurses
attitudes towards older people's nursing 56
commitment of 116
as front-line role models 60
role of in older people's nursing 57
nursing
as caring 102, 130
complexity of 47
definitions 48
influence of other disciplines on 49
nature of 46–7
sources of knowledge in 47–9
nursing assessment see assessment of patients
nursing-home sector 67
nursing models 91, 92, 107–8, 117–22
and nursing practice 118–21, 123

nursing practice 25, 46–7
  gap between theory and 25, 27,
    29, 30, 32, 33–4, 38, 50, 113, 122
  and nursing models 118–21, 123
  principles underpinning good
    128
Nursing Standard 114
nursing theory 25–51, 61, 107, 122
  definitions 28
  grand 27–8, 32, 40, 117, 120, 123,
    136
  language of 122
  levels of 31–3
  logical positivist perspective 28
  middle-range theories 33, 109,
    121, 136
  and practice gap 25, 27, 29, 30,
    32, 33–4, 38, 50, 113, 122
  and technical rationality model
    29–31
nursing therapeutics 94–101
  elimination care 96–7
  hygiene care 94–6
  medication and pain control 98–9
  nutritional care 97–8
  preventative and safety issues
    100–1
Nursing Times 114
nurturing aspects, of nursing care
  79, 81
nutritional care 97–8, 99

O'Brian, B. 86–7
observational studies 12–14
older people
  as an asset to the community 70
  experiences of treatment 58
  policies for improving lives of
    65–6
  sectors involved in long-term
    management of 69, 69
older people's nursing 52–4
  nurses' attitudes towards 56
  nurse's role 57

traditional 54–8
uniqueness of 122
on-the-spot experimenting 123, 135
open visiting policy 108
Opportunity Age 132

pain control 98–9
paradigm cases 35, 36, 37, 97, 99
patient-centred care see person-
  centred care
Peplau's exposition of nursing 32
perceptual awareness 35
person-centred care 52–3, 54, 56, 57,
  108–9, 114, 115, 117, 121–2, 129,
  133
personal knowledge 35, 37, 43, 82,
  87, 89, 99
personalisation 82
phenomenological aspects 32
physical activity 127
Polanyi, M. 44, 95
'Poor Law nurses' 54
positivism 30–1, 37
power
  and knowledge 104
practical knowledge 35–6, 39, 95, 97
practical wisdom 2, 39–41, 76, 82
practice theory 9, 26, 33–7, 44–5,
  136
  as descriptive theory 45
  developing of through older
    people's nursing 111
  as factor-isolating 45–6
  informal see informal practice
    theory
practitioner-based research 136
preventative issues 100–1
primary care 60, 132
  aim of new roles in 132
  older people's nursing in 70–2, 71
Primary Care Trusts 60
proactive approaches 66, 68
professional knowledge 34
Professional Nurse 114

professionals
    common characteristics shared
        by 34
propositional knowledge 99
PubMed 20
Pursey, A. 56

qualitative research 10, 11, 16, 111
quality of life, main building blocks
    for 132

reactive model 66
Recipe for Care – Not a Single
    Ingredient, A 67–8, 130–1
records, nursing 119–20
Redfern, S. 105, 112–13
Reed, J. 32, 107, 120, 121
reflection 41–3
reflection in and on action 43–6, 91,
    107, 123, 124, 135, 136
reflective cycle 43, *44*
reflective practice 26
reflexivity, researcher 16–17
rehabilitation 67, 88, 97, 101
relationship-centred care 53, 129 *see*
    also nurse–patient relationship
research methodology 9–24
    categorising the data 17–19
    comparing findings with nursing
        literature 19–20
    data collection methods 11–12
    ethical issues 10–11
    factor isolation 20–3, *22*
    field notes 15
    identifying relationships in the
        data 23
    interviews of nurses 13, 14–15
    nurse profile 12
    observations 12–14
    researcher reflexivity 16–17
    sampling decision 11–12
risk assessment 106–7, 108
rituals, and nursing 48–9
Robbins, I. 32, 107, 120

Rogers, M. E. 32
Rolfe, G. 40, 97
Roper, N. 91, 96, 107, 119, 120, 121
Ross, F. 112–13
Royal College of Nursing 57, 108,
    128
Ryle, G. 36

safety issues 100–1
sampling decisions 11–12
Schon, D. 26, 30, 34, 42, 43, 87, 91,
    95, 98, 99, 112, 116, 123, 124
scientific nursing 112–13
scientific positivist research 112, 124
self-care 60, 69, 76, 81, 89, 96, 101
senses framework 53–4, 129
Silverman, D. 12
Smith, C. 93, 103, 107
social care 59, 69, 132
somology 85
staff shortages 135
Stenhouse, L. 38
subjectivity 123–4
Sure Start to Later Life, A 126–7
Sweden 56

tacit knowledge 44, 89, 95
Taylor, C. 119
teamwork 94
technical rationality 29–31, 91, 112,
    120, 123, 136
theoretical knowledge 112
'theories in action' 121, 122
'theories in use' 42
theory
    informal *see* informal theory
    nursing *see* nursing theory
    and practice 38, 124
    see also practice theory
therapeutic bath 48–9
therapeutic care 76, 121, 128
therapeutics, nursing *see* nursing
    therapeutics
'total nursing care' 87, 103

Transcultural Care Theory 32
Tudor-Hart, J. 56–7

Usher, R. 29–30, 40, 46, 112, 116, 124

visiting policy 108

Walsh, M. 49
wards, hospital 74–7
    nurse-managed beds 75

nurses as key figures in overall
    management of 74–5, 113–14
    research study 74
Webster, G. 28
wellbeing, patient
    promoting of 46, 47, 66, 130
Wells, T. J. 55
Wittgenstein, L. 115–16
Wolf, Z. R. 48, 49
Wrubel, J. 33, 83, 121

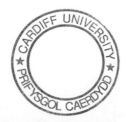